"'Hallelujah! Halleluhjah!' I said to myself over and over again as I read Laura's new book. Finally, *at last*, here is a book that speaks the truth about how so often women have taken on the male experience of Yoga, without understanding our own needs and energies. Laura has given voice to the power and deep goodness of the feminine in the world of Yoga.

Thank you, Laura, for this revelatory, insightful, fascinating, and beautiful book. A must read for those women who practice Yoga, as well as for those who don't."

~ Judith Hanson Lasater, Ph.D., P.T., and author of nine books on Yoga, including *Restore and Rebalance: Yoga for Deep Relaxation*

"Laura has given us a great gift through the birthing of *Moon Salutations*! As we align with the moon's feminine principles, we enhance the dynamic power women naturally embody, propelling us into an era where kindness, love and compassion, high feminine values, reign supreme."

~ Nischala Joy Devi, author, *The Healing Path of Yoga*, *The Secret Power of Yoga* and *The Namaste Effect*

"A great book that will help women to support and nourish themselves through menstruation, pregnancy, childbirth, menopause and simply being a woman. Laura provides guidelines for practice and the history of both Sun and Moon Salutations to reinforce the power of women and Yoga. With all good wishes for this book's success!"

~ Angela Farmer, cofounder of Yoga from the Inner Body

"A wise, full moon of a book. I had to stop, cheeks wet, remembering the transformative experience of practicing the Moon Salutation. I literally jumped from my chair to try it again, inspired anew by Cornell's stories and evocative descriptions. *Moon Salutations* will be a source of healing, acceptance and transformation for countless women who discover it on their path."

~ Amy Weintraub, Founder of LifeForce Yoga and author of *Yoga for Depression* and *Yoga Skills for Therapists*

"The very practices we need to remind us that the moon is half of who we are. Laura Cornell offers a corrective to the historical exclusion of women in Yoga and offers a path forward for feminine centered Yoga practice. I love this book!"
~ Cyndi Lee, author of *Yoga Body, Buddha Mind*

"A masterpiece of Yogic insight. This book delicately balances the personal with the calls and screams and songs of the universe and the universal. Daily practice of the Moon Salutation breaks down habits of negativity, empowering both women and men to become tenders and menders, no longer victimized by generations of societal and in some cases personal abuse."
~ Christopher Key Chapple, Ph.D., Director, M.A. in Yoga Studies Loyola Marymount and author of *Yoga and the Luminous: Patañjali's Spiritual Path to Freedom*

"A beautiful weaving of stories, yogic truth-telling, inspiration, and love. The Sun Salutation and hidden masculine values have long dominated Yoga and this book brings needed balance by reinstating the moon to her rightful place. Thank you Laura!"
~ Camille Maurine, author of *Meditation Secrets for Women*

"Laura Cornell is a stand-out voice and remarkable teacher in the area of Yoga and women's empowerment. Her cutting-edge wisdom is to be devoured. This book is no exception."
~ Rachael Jayne Groover, Creator of Art of Feminine Presence and author of *Powerful and Feminine*

"A gorgeous read... filled with generosity of spirit, understanding, and compassion. A visionary book that needed to be written for a long time, and I can't imagine anyone better to have done it."
~ Esther Wyss-Flamm, Ph.D., Mind-Body Coach for Women and Founder, Women's Leadership Institute

"What a wonderful gift! I love what you have written and will use your book in both my own practice and my teaching."
~ Deva Parnell, senior Kripalu Yoga teacher and co-creator of the Moon Salutation

MOON SALUTATIONS

Women's Journey Through Yoga to Healing, Power, and Peace

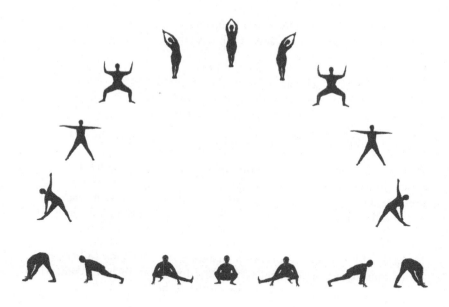

Laura Cornell, Ph.D.

Divine Feminine Yoga
Pleasant Hill, California

Moon Salutations: Women's Journey Through Yoga to Healing,
Power, and Peace

Copyright © 2019 by Laura Cornell. All rights reserved.
Printed in the United States of America.

Divine Feminine Yoga LLC
Pleasant Hill, CA 94523

First Edition
ebook ISBN: 978-1-7333923-1-0
Print ISBN: 978-1-7333923-0-3
First printing November 2019

Library of Congress Control Number:2019914592

The content of this book is for general instruction only. Each person's physical, emotional, and spiritual condition is unique. The instruction in this book is not intended to replace or interrupt the reader's relationship with a physician or other mental health professional. Please consult your doctor for matters pertaining to your specific health.

Cover Design by: Debbie O'Byrne
Layout Design by: www.JetLaunch.net
Back Cover Photo by: Jessica Hadari
Cover Model: Maria Arvayo

For Mom, who loves me now more than ever.
I see you blessing all who read this book.

CONTENTS

DREAM OF A FIELD OF LIGHT

I am driving home at night with my parents when we come upon the cornfield near our house. From the bottom of the hill it looks as if the rising ground is lit brightly from many houses and street lamps. I am surprised at the light, and I ask my mom, "They can't have built a city there, can they?"

As we come up over the ridge I see that the light is coming from the earth itself and from the many flowers growing unevenly around the field. The flowers are mostly weeds with some marigolds and sunflowers, and all are glowing brightly, giving off light.

In the back of the field a group of women dance in a circle with flowing arm movements. The women are larger than life in shining robes with long sleeves and flares at the cuffs and hem. A source of light stands at the center of the circle. I am in awe. ~ From my Journal, April 14, 1990

This dream came to me as a source of hope during one of the darkest periods of my life. I was in my mid-20s and had just been rejected from UC Berkeley, the graduate school of my choice. I wasn't sure what was next for me or how to pursue my career.

Worse still, I was in the middle of a super-bumpy dialogue with my parents. I had told first my mom and then my dad about the incest I had experienced with him. The gut-wrenching discomfort of that process is hard to put into words, even 30 years later. I was breaking family taboos on many levels ~ in speaking about sex, speaking about having been abused, and telling secrets my father had kept from my mother.

This dialogue with my parents was so draining and depleting that I came down with pneumonia the day after we had family therapy. At the time of this dream two months later, I was still recovering my strength.

This dream came as a profound gift. Confused about my direction in life, worried about my health, and feeling unsure in relation to my parents, the dream was a clear sign that my connection with the divine was alive and well. Despite the challenging circumstances of my life, here was a symbol of hope and healing.

It would be several more years before I received the gift of Yoga in my life to soothe and heal my frayed nervous system and to change the course of my life. But the signs of my own awakening divinity were already present. I felt a profound connection to nature ~ Mother Earth embracing and welcoming me. I felt the healing power of the women's circles in which I was participating.[1]

As this dream showed me, my journey was well in motion.

---

1. Many of these were circles that I met through Quakers. I spent 20 years worshiping with Friends, another source of strength and growth for me.

INTRODUCTION

1

UNDERSTANDING THE MOON SALUTATION

In the late 1980s, around the same time I was dreaming of shimmering women flowing in a circle, a group of senior female Yoga teachers in the Berkshire Mountains of Massachusetts was experimenting with new sequences of poses for women. These women were full-time residents at the Kripalu Center for Yoga and Health and had been living and breathing Yoga for many years.

The practice of Yoga poses they were being taught and were passing on to others wasn't well known at that time, having been brought to the United States not much more than 20 or 30 years earlier. Even less well known was how Yoga poses might need to differ for women. As the feminist movement swirled around them, these women couldn't help but notice that all the gurus were male, and that the physical and energetic practices they were being given felt oriented more toward men's bodies than women's bodies.

Among many other practices, they were taught the Sun Salutation, arguably the most well-known sequence of poses in modern Yoga. According to popular legend, the Sun Salutation was originally practiced both as a morning prayer to the sun and as physical and spiritual preparation for warriors. Based on a series of deep backward and forward bends, the Sun Salutation warms and energizes the body, giving an overall stretch to the major muscle groups.

Yet there are times in women's lives when the Sun Salutation may not be appropriate. For many women, the Sun Salutation as a whole is too heating during menstruation and menopause and should be practiced gently or not at all. Several of its postures are contraindicated for pregnancy, as they could injure either fetus or mother.

To complement and balance the Sun Salutation, these senior female teachers created the Moon Salutation, a flow of Yoga postures designed to support and nourish a woman's body. The Moon Salutation cools and calms the nervous system and includes several of the most beneficial postures for pregnancy, menstruation, and menopause. It is also a side-bending and squatting sequence, stretching and engaging muscles not affected by the Sun Salutation.

The women first presented their new sequence in 1988 as part of a new five-day intensive program "Women and Yoga." Megha Nancy Buttenheim, one of the co-creators of the Moon Salutation, tells the story in this way:

> We were asking, "How can we create a gentle experience that's more moon-based, more flowing, and something that would be wonderful for menstruation and menopause?" Women and Yoga was a prayer and the Moon Salutation was a moving celebration of that prayer.

Because the Moon Salutation orients the body sideways (rather than front to back) it is perfectly suited to practicing in a circle or facing a partner, opening us to relationship and community in our Yoga practice. Its earthy squats help us to feel grounded and open to emotions. Moon Salutations may be practiced at any time, but are especially soothing in the evening and especially celebratory on full or new moons.

If you are new to Moon Salutations, I can tell you you're in for a treat. Here are some of the benefits you can expect from this sequence:

- You will feel your heart open through Crescent Moon Poses.

- You will feel empowered through the Goddess Squat.

- You will feel connected to the earth through Lunge and Side Lunge Poses.

- Your body will be strengthened and stretched through side-bending, lunging, forward-bending, and squatting.

If you are a beginner to Yoga, remember to go easy as you start. You may want to show this book to your Yoga teacher and ask her or him to guide you through the poses one-by-one over a period of weeks before you attempt putting them together in a flow. I also include a gentle version in Chapter 9 that you can practice right out of the box from day one, even as a beginner, and even if you have stiff hips or knees or are in a chair.

If you have come across a version of the Moon Salutation in the past that was too difficult for you, take heart. This book includes versions that are do-able by beginners and experienced practitioners alike, including full circular Moon Salutations that are more accessible for many by using high lunges rather than low lunges.

Some of you may be experienced Yoga teachers or practitioners yearning to find a feminine voice and a feminine perspective on Yoga. To you I say, welcome, you're in the right place! There is much to learn about the vital history of women in Yoga, and the Moon Salutation is an excellent starting place.

2

MY STORY

Immediately after I became a Yoga teacher in 1995, I began to include the Moon Salutation in my Yoga teaching, both in classes exclusively for women as well as in mixed-gender groups. I will often lead it in retreats. When I show the Moon Salutation to women, I find there is an immediate sense of recognition, almost an "aha" experience. Demonstrating the salutation requires intense concentration and attention, making its practice in a group setting even more of an offering than when I am alone. In these moments I feel as though my personal identity as "Laura" fades somewhat, and I embody instead the universal feminine, the Goddess.

As we practice the Moon Salutation together, the whole group shares the sense of embodiment of the divine. We often practice in a circle, creating a sense of sacred ritual. Later, students report how significant this flow is to them. Many begin to practice it at home and to teach it to friends and family.

I was blessed to learn both the Sun and Moon Salutations from friends. When I first moved to California in 1988, a friend from college excitedly showed me a sequence of Yoga poses he had learned recently. I still remember his delight in teaching me the Sun Salutation, and his story of practicing three rounds each morning in his Santa Cruz backyard. As it turned out, this was my first, albeit brief, introduction to the modern practice of Yoga. I practiced the Sun Salutation for six years before another friend showed me the Moon Salutation, telling me its story as a Yoga flow created by and for women. I remember practicing this sequence facing her, our bodies mirroring each other as we moved between the poses, and connecting hands as we bowed our heads in the Side Lunge.

Less than a year later I attended the Women and Yoga Program at Kripalu, just before my Yoga Teacher Training. The Women and Yoga program provided a powerful container for gestating the stories of our lives. We shared personal anecdotes, delved deeply into the Moon Salutation, and engaged in practices that were at times nourishing, at times vigorous, but always affirming of our feminine selves. Practicing Yoga in this circle of women connected me to a new sense of purpose and meaning.

I have found the Moon Salutation to be an ideal form for me. In my personal Yoga practice, I am a *bhakti yogini*, one who grows through cultivating devotion. Thus the salutations are important for me because they accentuate the devotional aspect of the practice. Further, as a woman in this patriarchal culture, I have needed to recover from society's warping effects on my development. While the embodied practice of Yoga helps me to re-inhabit and love my physical form, the Moon Salutation in particular enables me to embrace its feminine aspects. Through the Moon Salutation, I feel the beauty and power of my feminine being, I express gratitude and connection to Mother Earth, and I create a healing community with other women.

I've been a Yoga teacher for 24 years. I've led more than 1,000 classes, workshops, and retreats, including more than 40 retreats for women only. I've led the Moon Salutation to thousands of women and men in groups large and small. I've taught toddlers through frail elderly, and everyone in between. Through all of this, the Moon Salutation has been a faithful companion, not always in the foreground, but always nearby and in my mind as a familiar friend.

The Moon Salutation has been one of my best tools for healing my own trauma. It has nourished my body and invited me to love myself as a woman more deeply than I ever thought possible. It has connected me with other women in circles of all sizes and helped me to remember the wisdom of my grandmothers and of this blessed planet.

3

HOW TO READ THIS BOOK

More than just presenting a sequence of poses, this book is a story ~ a story of lives, both of the women who created this flow and those of us who have lived it since. It is the story of how this Yoga sequence has touched us, opened us and healed us, and of the groups and places along the way where we have experienced it.

I wrote the first edition of this book 20 years ago as my master's thesis while a graduate student at the California Institute of Integral Studies.[2] I conducted interviews with more than 30 Yoga teachers across the United States including the women who were the co-creators of the Moon Salutation. I also went deep into my own experience of this flow ~ meditating, moving through the poses, journaling, teaching, and listening to my muse. Before holding any of the interviews, I condensed my experiential process into a meditative poem to accompany the Moon Salutation, found in Chapter 15.

This completely revised and updated version includes even more personal stories and anecdotes, more variations than the original version, and more about a woman's journey of healing from all forms of loss and trauma. For this revised and updated version, I sought additional interviews and contributions. I give a deep bow to the many women and men who contributed their stories for both the original and this expanded version. The contributors are listed in the back of the book and also where quoted.

---

2. Laura Cornell. *The Moon Salutation: Expression of the Feminine in Body, Psyche, Spirit* (Emeryville, CA: Yogeshwari Arts, 2000).

Chapters 5 and 6 discuss the origins and mythology of the Sun Salutation as well as the historical background of women in the practice of Yoga. These chapters set the stage for understanding the significance of a salutation created as a response to the Sun Salutation and to the male orientation of Yoga in general. Next in Chapter 7, I explore the beginnings of the Moon Salutation, showing how the creativity and inner awareness fostered by the Kripalu Community of the late 1980s provided fertile ground for its birth. Chapter 8 discusses the poses of the Moon Salutation in detail, considering both physiological and psychological aspects. Chapters 9 through 11 give many possible variations, ranging from gentle versions for beginners or those with stiff hips and knees to the full circular Moon Salutation and beyond, for those desiring more challenge.

Later chapters of the book unfold 13 key features of the Moon Salutation:

1. It centers and grounds us. (Chapter 12)

2. It invokes celebration on the full moon and quiet on the new moon. (Chapters 13 and 14)

3. It is more cooling energetically than the Sun Salutation. (Chapter 16)

4. It nourishes the hips and pelvis. (Chapter 16)

5. It awakens spherical consciousness, not linear consciousness. (Chapter 16)

6. It honors menstruation, pregnancy, and menopause. (Chapters 17, 18, and 20)

7. It beckons us to love our bodies. (Chapter 21)

8. It invites us into a circle of women. (Chapter 22)

9. It helps us heal from sexual trauma. (Chapter 23)

10. It balances upper and lower chakras. (Chapter 25)

11. It integrates opposites while encouraging us to move beyond them. (Chapters 24 and 26)

12. It calls men to honor the feminine principle. (Chapter 27)

13. It unfolds peace. (Chapters 28 and 29)

ALL ARE INVITED

You don't need to identify as a woman to learn this flow. For example, some men practice the Moon Salutation every full moon in order to celebrate the cycles of nature. Others practice it to honor the divine feminine in their lives or because it is such a powerful physical, psychological, and spiritual counterbalance to the Sun Salutation. Moon Salutations may be practiced in mixed-gender groups, women's groups, men's groups, or by oneself, and by anyone of any gender including non-binary or gender-non-conforming.

OTHER MOON SALUTATIONS

As practice of the Sun Salutation became widespread in India starting in the 1920s and beyond, it was only natural that wise teachers would look for ways to cool its inherent heat. Swami Satyananda Saraswati of the Bihar School of Yoga created such a Moon Salutation, a modified, somewhat more cooling version of the Sun Salutation.[3] Following his lead, others also teach a similar flow.[4] Just to be clear, this slight modification of the Sun Salutation is fundamentally different from what I am referring to in this book, which is a side-bending and squatting sequence.

Ultimately, a Moon Salutation is a greeting and an acknowledgement of peace, gentleness, and wholeness. It is a way of living, not limited to any particular Yoga flow. A Moon Salutation

3. See Swami Satyananda Saraswati, *Asana, Pranayama, Mudra, Bandha,* (Bihar: India, Yoga Publications Trust). The flow begins by stepping the left foot back (instead of the right) on the first round in order to stimulate the *ida* (lunar or cooling) channel in the body. Then after Lunge Pose the arms are taken up overhead with back knee remaining on the ground. Mantras to the Divine Feminine are to be said along with the movements. Swami Satyananda refers to his sequence using the Sanskrit translation *Chandra Namaskar,* but the meaning is the same.

4. Dr. Vasant Lad and Shiva Rea are two examples.

is any time we stop to feel the moon in our heart, to see her presence with us in the sky, or simply anytime we smile at the moon inwardly and feel her smile back. Moon Salutations honor women's bodies and women's lives.

This book is a tapestry, a weaving together of journal entries, conversations, poems, and stories from friends, students, clients, and colleagues gathered over the last two-and-a-half decades of my life. Most of all, this book is a journey of the soul ~ my journey, other practitioners' journeys, and a journey I invite you, the reader, to share with us. We invite you into our circle.

4
A GIFT FOR YOU

This book tells a story, but there is so much more to experience. Yoga is meant to be lived. I've created videos, a downloadable meditation audio, mini-poster and more to accompany this book, and will host videos from some of our contributors. Please visit www.MoonSalutations.com for these resources and more.

Please visit www.MoonSalutations.com.

PART ONE: WHY WE NEED MOON SALUTATIONS

5

THE SUN SALUTATION ~ MYTHS AND TRADITIONS

When I admire the wonders of a sunset or the beauty of the moon, my soul expands in worship of the creator.

~ Mahatma Gandhi

In order to understand the Moon Salutation, we first need to understand the Sun Salutation, a hallmark of contemporary Yoga ~ the most familiar and frequently taught sequence of poses. The Sun Salutation carries a mystique that often extends beyond what may be established through scholarly means. However, the mythological story of its origin gives fascinating insight into its meaning for practitioners today.

The Sun Salutation is said to have been taught to Rama to enable him to succeed in the great epic battle described in the ancient Sanskrit tale of the *Ramayana*. Thus, the Sun Salutation is a spiritual tool for warriors. The following explanation is from Apa Pant, son of the king of the Indian state of Aundh, who is credited with popularizing the Sun Salutation in the first half of the 20th Century:

It is said that when Rama faced Ravana on the battlefield, he received the great knowledge of the technique of Surya Namaskars *[Sun Salutations] from the sage Vishvamitra. It was this knowledge that enabled Rama to endure the strain of battle against Ravana, an enemy far superior to him in armored strength. Those who seek good health, greater equilibrium of mind, conquest over slothfulness and tiredness should certainly practice these exercises.*[5]

The concept of battle may be understood symbolically as well as literally, referring to the many daily challenges we face. According to Pant, the Sun Salutation gives its practitioners health, vitality, and assistance in the battle against inner and outer enemies.

The battle between Rama and Ravana in the *Ramayana* corresponds with Joseph Campbell's description of the Hero's Journey, which Campbell describes as the archetypal human journey, involving an adventurous struggle for identity and self-definition. The journey includes "a separation from the world, a penetration to some sense of power, and a life-enhancing return."[6] The hero meets with perils and obstacles as well as good fortune and helpers along the way. If the Sun Salutation was a magical aid for Rama in his Hero's Journey, so too can it be a magical tool in our human quest for identity.

This interpretation corresponds with my experience of the Sun Salutation. Each time the heart reaches upward in a backbend, there is a sense of opening to life's challenges and facing them courageously. Each time the body bends forward, there is a feeling of surrender and acceptance of divine grace, as when Rama receives guidance from his teacher, Vishvamitra. In the lunge, there is a sense of stepping forward into action. And in the final standing pose, there is peace and accomplishment. The battle has been won, the enemy faced, and the warrior arrives home transformed.

Daily prayers to the sun, which in some parts of India include multiple full-body prostrations, have been common since Vedic times of several millennia BCE. The most familiar Vedic *mantra* (prayer), the *Gayatri Mantra*, is dedicated to the sun as a spiritual symbol of radiance and power. Yet, although solar prayers were known at the time of the *Ramayana* and before, the age of the Sun Salutation as we know it today is difficult to determine.

---

5. Apa Pant, *Surya Namaskars: An Ancient Indian Exercise,* 3rd ed. (Bombay: Orient Longman, 1989), 3.

6. Joseph Campbell, *The Hero with a Thousand Faces* (Princeton, NJ: Princeton University Press, 1968), 35.

The classical works on Hatha Yoga do not mention any standing flows. These works are primarily concerned with seated meditation postures, *pranayama* (breathing practices), *mudras* (energy seals), and *bandhas* (locks). The Sun Salutation in its current sequence and makeup of postures seems most likely to have developed from the intermixing of ancient solar worship with modern influences.[7]

In the early 20th Century, the Sun Salutation was considered separate from Yoga; practicing it as part of Yoga was said to be "ill-informed" and "prohibited."[8] Shri Yogendra, who founded the first modern postural Yoga school in Bombay in 1918, asserts:

> Surya Namaskars *or prostrations to the sun ~ a form of gymnastics attached to the sun worship in India ~ indiscriminately mixed up with the Yoga physical training by the ill-informed are definitely prohibited by the authorities.*[9]

Gradually, however, the Sun Salutation became so popular and well integrated into modern postural Yoga that the memory of any non-yogic or Western influence was erased.

The tradition of Ashtanga Yoga asserts that the Sun Salutation is recorded in an ancient text, the *Yoga Kurunta*, purported to be at least 1,000 years old, and taught to K. Pattabhi Jois, Ashtanga

---

7. Georg Feuerstein, "The Origins of the Sun Salutation," *Yoga World: International Newsletter for Yoga Teachers and Students* 8 (1999); see also Mark Singleton, *Yoga Body: The Origins of Modern Posture Practice* (New York: Oxford University Press, 2010). During the colonial period, the royal palaces were generous patrons of a wide range of intellectual and physical culture. Hatha Yoga mingled with classical Indian sports such as wrestling and with the newly popular British sports of gymnastics and bodybuilding. This led to the assimilation of new postures into Yoga, as well as new syntheses and sequences of postures. The series of postures known as *Surya Namaskar* (Sun Salutation) was first recorded in the 1880s in the *Shri Tattvanidhi*, commissioned by the King of Mysore, and including a wide-ranging compilation of physical and spiritual practices known in South India at the time.

8. Mark Singleton, *Yoga Body: The Origins of Modern Posture* (New York: Oxford University Press, 2010), 180.

9. Shri Yogendra. *Yoga Asanas Simplified.* 1st ed., 1928 (Mumbai: The Yoga Institute, 2006), 99.

Yoga's founder, by his teacher, Shri T. Krishnamacharya. There is good evidence however, that this is not actually an ancient document but was written by Krishnamacharya himself, as was at least one other text he had attributed to ancient sources.[10]

Writer and teacher Anne Cushman gives a humorous account of the flavor of this debate. While Krishnamacharya is said to have unearthed the palm-leafed *Yoga Kurunta* in a Calcutta library, reportedly it was eaten by ants; not one copy was ever found.[11] According to Yoga scholar Mark Singleton, Jois was exposed to the Sun Salutation while studying under Krishnamacharya at the Palace of Mysore in the 1930s, where Yoga classes took place just down the hall from (then completely distinct) Sun Salutation classes.

Scholarly debate continues about which poses were borrowed from whom, and which version was ancient or a modern amalgam. The more important question for us is: What is useful for our own bodies and our own healing? What brings our soul to a place of peace and growth?

Whatever the historical facts, the Sun Salutation transmits the energy of the Hero's Journey, giving practitioners the strength and power to surmount obstacles and work toward positive self-definition. It carries the solar qualities of vigor, determination, and persistence, as well as humility and surrender. In contrast, the Moon Salutation enacts the journey of descent ~ sinking into the depths to discover one's creativity, the process of literal or metaphoric birth, just as the moon goes through dark phases and returns to its full brilliance.

Perhaps most importantly, in addition to understanding the gifts of the Sun Salutation for practitioners today, the story of how the Sun Salutation became integrated into 20th Century Yoga shows us also that Yoga is constantly evolving, growing from the needs of the people it serves. As was said of Krishnamacharya, "He was always innovating, always experimenting."[12] Great teachers draw on ancient wisdom but also constantly pay attention to what is needed by their students ~ and by the times at hand.

---

10. Singleton, *Yoga Body*, 185.

11. Anne Cushman, "New Light on Yoga," *Yoga Journal* 147 (July/August, 1999), 46.

12. Singleton, *Yoga Body*, 187.

6

A BRIEF HISTORY OF WOMEN'S EXCLUSION FROM YOGA

*The criticism of women in the orthodox Sanskrit literature ...
is indicative of the popular inhibition which took its ugly form
that a woman is a useless appendage to a spiritually healthy man.*

~ Shri Yogendra, Founder, The Yoga Institute[13]

*Women, when compared to men, have a special right to practice
Yoga. This is because it is women who are responsible for the
continuity of the lineage.*

~ T. Krishnamacharya, widely considered the
"father" of modern Yoga.[14]

The two quotes above, written at the cusp of Yoga's emergence into the modern era, are taken from two men who played foundational roles in establishing the Yoga we know today. Shri Yogendra opened his Yoga Institute in 1918, the first postural Yoga school to include women, children, and all castes. Beginning in 1933, T. Krishnamacharya taught at the

---

13. Sitadevi Yogendra, *Yoga Physical Education for Women* (Santacruz East: The Yoga Institute, 1988). This quote is from the Introduction to the book, p. 17.

14. From the *Yoga Rahasya*, verse 1:14. by T. Krishnamacharya, quoted in Eric Shaw, 2016 "Krishnamacharya's Yoga Rahasya," http://www.sutrajournal. com/krishnamacharyas-Yoga-rahasya-by-eric-shaw, retrieved on January 11, 2019.

Palace of the King of Mysore. Several of his students went on to popularize Yoga worldwide, including B. K. S. Iyengar, K. Pattabhi Jois, and Krishnamacharya's son, T. K. V. Desikachar.

After multiple requests and only at the behest of his patron, the Mysore King, Krishnamacharya finally accepted the Russian actress and dancer Indra Devi as his student in 1938.[15] He was widely criticized for including a foreign woman in his otherwise all-male classes, although he had been teaching female family members before that.

When Krishnamacharya wrote of the need to include women in Yoga, he spoke from his own experience as an adept yogi who later became a husband and father of two daughters, his first-born children. He spoke from his heart, but against millennia of orthodox tradition that had excluded women from advanced spiritual practice, including the traditional forms of Yoga and meditation. Krishnamacharya also came to believe in his later life that if Yoga were not taught to all peoples and especially to women it was likely to die out.[16]

The modern era brought massive shifts to millennia-old practices such as Yoga. The value of equality meant that it was no longer acceptable for women to be excluded or for the practice to be available only to upper-caste Brahmins. Scientific inquiry meant that poses were studied for their physiological effects. While women were initially subject to general restrictions such as to avoid Yoga during "menstruation and advanced pregnancy,"[17] modifications as needed for various poses came to be accepted, and we came to realize that modified Yoga at these times was highly beneficial.

As ideas spread more rapidly, cross-fertilization of practices increased. Secularization meant that esoteric or religiously embedded practices were now taught in simpler form, apart from their earlier cultural context. Perhaps most importantly, practices previously reserved only for a select few became widely available to the masses. These big changes gave us contemporary Yoga.

---

15. Devi later became the first woman to popularize Yoga worldwide.

16. T. K. V. Desikachar, quoted in Eric Shaw, 2016 "Krishnamacharya's Yoga Rahasya," http://www.sutrajournal.com/krishnamacharyas-Yoga-rahasya-by-eric-shaw, retrieved on January 11, 2019.

17. Sitadevi Yogendra, *Yoga: Physical Education for Women*, 13.

As Yoga developed over millennia in India, women undoubtedly participated in its practice and evolution, but they were excluded from its more visible and dominant forms. In a very few of the ancient texts, women were initiated into the teachings of Yoga by their husbands or brothers.[18] In these texts, women are portrayed as being just as intelligent, inquiring, and spiritually qualified as men.[19]

Primarily however, women were expected to be devoted wives and mothers,[20] and to carry out home-based rituals for the well-being of the family.[21] They woke early before dawn to perform prayers and housework, continued with required periods of devotion and work throughout the day, and often spent evenings in even more devotional practices such as listening to the *Puranas* (stories of deities) or participating in an extensive array of religious festivals.

Another role available to women was that of *devadasi,* meaning "wife of God." These women were temple dancers who literally married God. They were the best educated and most independent women in the culture. Living collectively in the temples, they owned their own property, studied scripture, and practiced spiritual arts such as dance, music, and lovemaking. Sadly, during the colonial period the British saw these women only as prostitutes and their participation in temple life was outlawed. Western prudishness very nearly obliterated a long-standing tradition that was rich in women's spiritual experience. Contemporary

18. Parvati was initiated by Shiva, Gargi (sometimes called Maitreyi) by Yajnavalkya.

19. For example, Muktabai, Jnaneshwar's sister, was initiated by him into Nath Yoga in the 13th Century, and is said to have attained the divine body (*divya sharira*)

20. Julia Leslie, *Roles and Rituals for Hindu Women* (Cranbury, NJ: Associated University Presses, 1991).

21. Elinor Gadon, "Sanctifying the Home: The Ritual Art of the Women of Bengal," in *Sacred Dimensions of Women's Experience*, ed. Elizabeth D. Gray (Wellesley, MA: Roundtable Press, 1988); Elinor Gadon, "The Hindu Goddess Shashti: Protector of Women and Children," in *From the Realm of the Ancestors: An Anthology in Honor of Marija Gimbutas*, ed. Marija Gimbutas and Joan Marler (Manchester, CT: Knowledge Ideas & Trends, 1997); and Pupul Jayakar, *The Earth Mother: Legends, Ritual Arts, and Goddesses of India* (New York: Harper and Row, 1990).

Indian classical dance grew from an attempt to rescue a part of the devadasi lineage. But this newly sanitized art form eliminated much of the breadth and cultural context of women's earlier temple experience.[22]

A few other women stepped outside of tradition to become spiritual renunciates. These women longed to know divinity and merge with it fully. Their worship primarily took the form of ecstatic devotion (*bhakti*) and their poetry became widely known. Muktabai, Mirabai, and Lal ded Yogeshwari (Lalleshwari) are a few examples.

Despite women's clear spiritual interest and capacity, India remained a solidly patriarchal and class-stratified culture. Women, along with those in the untouchable caste, were forbidden from participating in *Brahmin* (upper caste) rituals or from reciting the Vedic *mantras*. For example, the *Gayatri Mantra* described in Chapter 5 was not to be recited by women.

Common belief was that liberation was possible only in a male body. Adi Shankaracharya, the great teacher of Advaita Vedanta who lived in the eighth or ninth century C.E., wrote that it was better to have been born a man than a woman.[23] Tradition held that a woman needed to be reborn in a future lifetime as a lower-caste man, and after multiple rebirths be reborn as a Brahmin male, and then and only then could she be initiated into spiritual practice.

Women's role in Hatha Yoga itself is difficult to ascertain. Some notable teachers hold that women were instrumental in the early, shamanic rituals that led to its creation.[24] Yet it is clear that for several millennia at least, women's participation in orthodox Yoga was strongly suppressed.

---

22. See Frédérique A. Marglin, *Wives of the God-king: The Rituals of the Devadasis of Puri* (New York, NY: Oxford University Press., 1985) and Jalaja Bonheim, *Aphrodite's Daughters: Women's Sexual Stories and the Journey of the Soul* (New York: Simon & Schuster, 1997) for more information on this tradition and its demise.

23. Swami Satprakashananda, *The Goal and the Way: The Vedantic Approach to Life's Problems* (St. Louis, MO: The Vedanta Society of St. Louis, 1977), 51.

24. Vicki Noble. "The Double Goddess." Lecture given at the California Institute of Integral Studies, San Francisco, CA, March 10, 2000; and Angela Farmer. "Empowerment for Women through Yoga." Workshop given at Body/Mind/Spirit Yoga Journal Conference, Estes Park, CO, October 10, 1998.

Indeed, the texts most often pointed to as the classics of Hatha Yoga were created by and for men. These texts include the *Goraksha Paddhati*, the *Hatha Yoga Pradipika*, the *Gheranda Samhita*, and the *Siva Samhita*.[25] In describing physical Yoga postures such as Lion Pose (*Simhasana*) or Sage's Pose (*Siddhasana*), practitioners are told where to place the feet in relation to the male sexual organs. No corresponding female instructions are given.[26]

The body is also said to have nine openings or gates: eyes, ears, nostrils, mouth, urethra, and anus.[27] This typology excludes the vagina, a passageway central to a woman's body. In a very specific way then, female anatomy is not considered in the detailed instructions of these works.

It is important to remember, however, that written texts are not the definitive statement on the actual spiritual practice of a people. As noted above in relation to the village tradition of India, many vital spiritual currents are simply never written down. These include, most often, women's traditions and those of the non-dominant races and classes. Instead, these traditions are transmitted through home rituals, folk tales, folk art, lullabies, and other songs.

WESTERN WOMEN DECIPHERING CELIBACY

The fact that women were often excluded from the dominant streams of Yoga means that as it has come to the West, certain aspects of its practice in relation to women have been insufficiently understood by some teachers, and thus transmitted in ways that are incorrect, incomplete, or simply confusing to their female students.

One example of this confusion lies in the delicate topic of celibacy, or the conservation of sexual energy. The actual workings of celibacy (*brahmacharya*, or energy conservation) are complex

---

25. For some context as to the dates of these texts: *Goraksha Paddhati*: 12th or 13th century C.E.; *Hatha Yoga Pradipika*: 14th century C.E.; *Gheranda Samhita*: 17th century C.E.; and *Siva Samhita*: 17th or 18th century C.E.

26. See for example *Hatha Yoga Pradipika* II. 21, 22 and II. 35, 37

27. Georg Feuerstein, *The Yoga Tradition: Its History, Literature, Philosophy and Practice* (Prescott, AZ: Hohm Press, 1998), 534; and Satprakashananda, *The Goal and the Way*, 50.

and difficult to understand in a Western framework, where they are so easily conflated with various forms of repression. Still, celibacy has long been a central requirement for those desiring to enter the disciplined yogic path. Both Patanjali's *Yoga Sutras* and the *Bhagavad Gita* refer to it as fundamental.

Those living at the Kripalu Ashram in the 1970s, '80s, and up until 1994 were required to practice celibacy. But some women at Kripalu found the explanation given for brahmacharya confusing in relation to their bodies. They were told that conservation of semen was a primary reason for celibacy. Indeed, sublimation of semen is frequently referred to in the ancient texts as a benchmark of yogic achievement. Yet it is difficult for women to translate how this practice may be effected in our female bodies.

Deva Parnell, who was a senior teacher at Kripalu and co-creator of the Moon Salutation, explains the lack of a satisfying explanation for this practice for women:

> *The technology of Yoga was in sublimating the semen so that it would be transformed into* ojas *(sacred fluid) and that this would lead to enlightenment. There was a question in my mind about whether or not this was the same for women... [Our teacher's] response was that the female equivalent of semen was the sexual juice or lubricating fluid. I didn't buy that. I didn't think that came anywhere near as powerful as the sperm. What would be equivalent to sperm would be egg, and that we have no control over. [This question] was never clearly answered for me as a woman.*

And Deva wasn't the only woman who noticed this. Another woman who was a senior teacher at the time explained the female equivalent of losing ojas as the menstrual flow, also a confusing comparison for many women.

Tanya Davis (not her real name), a Kripalu resident at the time and later programs leader, recounted her experience in this way:

> *Some of us questioned what our teacher was saying about energy. He was always telling the men to bring the energy in and up. Specifically, he would refer to bringing the semen in and up, but he also meant it in general energetically. We asked him about this, but he never seemed to get it. He just*

didn't understand why we would ask if it was different for a woman.

The root of the confusion about energy is the Sanskrit word *bindu*, which means "semen" but also "seed" or "source." It is the bindu that according to the practice of brahmacharya is the source of precious alchemical transformations. If bindu means seed on a literal level, then is the female ovum equivalent to the seed? If so, it is clear that the release of this precious substance in women occurs independent of the sexual act. Is sexual activity thus less depleting for women because procreative substances are not lost? If so, then is celibacy more important on a physical level for men than women?

This question is not immaterial. It goes straight to a root issue, that of trust in the teacher and his or her teachings. If brahmacharya is given as an essential practice in spiritual awakening, and if the explanation for its practice feels relevant for the male body but confused in relation to the female, what is the female student to think? Can the female student fully trust the teachings of a male teacher deriving from a male lineage? Are his instructions to her based on correct knowledge of her female body or rather on knowledge of the male body simply extended to the female? Feminist thought in the fields of psychology and medicine has shown how the assumption of male as norm leads to diminished understanding of human nature and functioning; the male cannot be taken as norm for both sexes.

As women at Kripalu grappled with these questions of celibacy and with their own spiritual evolution, one answer that felt right for them as women was the concept of expansion. Tanya Davis shares the explorations she and her sisters were having, and an answer that made sense to her:

> I remember in particular one study group that I was in with an elder resident and one of my teachers. I remember us asking: What is our own spiritual evolution? If "in and up" doesn't feel right to us, then what does? She responded that it is about the energy expanding and opening, becoming more and more all-encompassing. That felt right to me. As women our spiritual evolution is about the constant expansion of energy and being with what is in the moment.

Given the previous emphasis on male experience, it is only natural that women in recent decades have felt the need to closely examine how Yoga conforms to a woman's body. What works and what doesn't? Where must adaptations be made or new elements added? And, even further, in what ways might a woman's unique consciousness, psychology, and spirituality inform the practice?

These questions have led to the expansion of Yoga in response to the needs of women. Rather than discrediting the validity of the practice, women have sought instead to make it broader and more flexible. Women seek a Yoga practice that is at times restorative and nourishing rather than vigorous and taxing, a practice that emerges from the inner wisdom of the body rather than being imposed by an external authority, and a practice that reaches out to embrace an ever-expanding, ever-widening consciousness rather than being uni-dimensional and uni-directional.

We need Moon Salutations because sun honoring was brought into the modern practice of postural Yoga, but moon honoring was not. We need Moon Salutations because the solar (heating) channel in our body needs to be balanced by the lunar (cooling) channel. We need Moon Salutations because women's bodies and physical requirements deserve to be honored and included in the full practice of Yoga. We need Moon Salutations to express and empower feminine spiritual experience.

7

THE BIRTH OF THE MOON SALUTATION

The Moon Salutation was birthed through an intuitive and collaborative process. This was not the work of any one woman, but rather of an informal group of women who shared their ideas and movement explorations with one another. These explorations in turn grew from the deeply embodied wisdom that Kripalu Yoga encouraged and developed in its students. In order to understand the birth of the Moon Salutation, it is necessary to first understand the uniquely supportive environment in which it gestated.

Kripalu Yoga developed in the early 1970s from the teachings of Amrit Desai, who had initially come to the United States from India to study art. Desai's Yoga teaching became highly popular, and a vibrant community of American seekers grew up around him. Here the ancient practices of Yoga ~ primarily Hatha Yoga, meaning postures and breath; Bhakti Yoga, or devotional worship; and Raja Yoga, or disciplined meditation ~ mixed with modern Western sensibilities, including an openness to change and new ideas (particularly non-Western and non-Christian), humanistic psychology, and later feminism and transpersonal psychology.

The intermingling of vital currents from East and West generated a tremendous spiritual energy and a rich brew for innovations in Yoga and personal growth. This intermixing of a variety of intellectual and physical currents had much in common with the global fusion that took place in the Indian royal palaces of the colonial period, a place where the Sun Salutation likely derived and where modern Yoga was supported.

While in India, Desai had studied Yoga under Swami Kripalvananda, a tantric adept who was well known and dearly beloved to the people of his native Gujarat. The ancient lineage of Swami Kripalvananda was based on the awakening of *kundalini*, the spiritual energy that lies dormant in every human being. The kundalini is known as a serpent lying coiled at the base of the spine. Its awakening leads to the complete transformation of one's being. This process is supported by an ethical and balanced lifestyle, by breathwork, Hatha Yoga, chanting, and meditation, and by receiving grace from a teacher, but ultimately it is less a set of practices than a complete surrender to the divine.[28]

As Kripalu Yoga evolved in the West, it came to be known as a "Yoga of the heart." According to an early student who preferred to remain anonymous, "Desai's teachings were always about love. He would say 'Move into love, don't move into fear.'" The word "*Kripalu*," taken from the name of Swami Kripalvananda, means "compassion" or "kindness."

In 1971, after visiting Swami Kripalvananda in India, Desai began to experience spontaneous posture flow. Here the body moves of its own accord while the mind remains in profound meditation. Such an occurrence is known as *pranotthana*, or extended flow of *prana*, life force.

Desai began to orient his teaching toward enabling his students to experience this awakening of prana. Harriet L. Russell (Bhumi), an early student of Desai and a co-creator of the Moon Salutation, shared with me the following story:

> *My spontaneous posture flow occurred up in a cabin. I was ready to go to bed when all of a sudden I had a very deep urge, as though a message were saying, "You must get up and do Yoga." I flowed through many postures for probably forty-five minutes. When it ended, I had a feeling of peace, as though I understood the universe. It was a very deep experience. I had been doing the same sequence of postures every day for eighteen months, a posture sequence that we*

---

28. See Stuart Sovatsky, *Words from the Soul: Time, East/West Spirituality, and Psychotherapeutic Narrative* (New York: State University of New York Press, 1998) for an excellent discussion of kundalini and the problematics of its oversimplification in American culture.

had developed at the ashram. When this prana flow came,
it was completely different poses; it was completely out of
sync. But my body had been prepared by the intensive prac-
tice I had been doing for so long.

Similarly, all of the women who created the Moon Salutation
drew from their personal experiences of many years of practice.

Kripalu Yoga came to place major emphasis on the emergence
of this prana flow. Shri Jnaneshvar refers to it as the "action of
the body in which reason takes no part and which does not
originate as an idea springing in the mind."[29] Student of Swami
Kripalvananda and Yoga scholar, Stuart Sovatsky, points out that
this opening of prana belongs to the "vast expanse of precursor
states" to kundalini awakening, but should not be confused with
that awakening itself.[30]

Because Kripalu Yoga so deeply honored the spiritual potential in
each individual, there was tremendous room for creativity. Students
of Desai developed a wide range of programs in Yoga, health, bodywork, and spiritual attunement for the many guests who visited
their retreat center. Out of the Kripalu community grew Phoenix
Rising Yoga Therapy, LifeForce Yoga for Depression, Integrative
Yoga Therapy, Kripalu YogaDance®, and Kripalu Bodywork. Rather
than being constrained to teach only in ways they had been taught,
Kripalu teachers were free to innovate based on inner wisdom.

The spontaneous movement approach of Kripalu Yoga was seen
by some as representing an openness to exploring the feminine
aspects of Yoga, which might have been more difficult in traditions where postures were more formalized. One early resident,
who preferred to remain anonymous, spoke about this space for
women's explorations:

The female energy at Kripalu has always been very strong,
so for that aspect to come forth [in special programs for
women and in the Moon Salutation] it didn't meet a lot of
resistance. Amrit himself had a very strong feminine aspect.
He was very soft in his way of teaching. Kripalu Yoga had

---

29. Shri Jnaneshvar, *Jnaneshwari*, trans. V. Pradhan (Albany, NY: State
University of New York Press, 1987), verse 51.

30. Sovatsky, *Words from the Soul*, 154.

started as a spontaneous prana flow, an essentially receptive experience.

The receptive process the residents were being taught led to an environment that was open to feminine innovations.

Women at Kripalu were also increasingly interested in exploring the feminine experience of Yoga as distinct from the masculine. Despite the respect for embodied wisdom that prevailed at Kripalu, many women were feeling the constraints of living within a male-dominated society and a male-dominated ashram. Megha Nancy Buttenheim, co-director of the first Women and Yoga program and a co-creator of the Moon Salutation, shared her concerns:

> *While most of those who practice Yoga in the United States are women, the tradition itself is highly male-dominated, and the ancient texts patriarchal. Women ran the ashram but there was always a male guru. They used to put a picture of Mary up at Christmas and I would ask, "Couldn't we just leave it up so that there would be something I could relate to?"*

The women of Kripalu in the 1980s began to explore ways in which traditional spiritual paths are rooted in patriarchal forms. Some of them researched the ancient Goddess traditions, drawing from books such as *The Chalice and The Blade*[31] and *The Feminine Face of God*[32] for inspiration.

A group of women began to experiment with a sequence of postures that would specifically honor women's bodies and rhythms. They wanted their new creation to complement and balance the Sun Salutation. And they wanted it to benefit women at all stages of their life cycle.

According to Deva Parnell, Senior Kripalu Yoga teacher and co-creator of the Moon Salutation:

---

31. Riane T. Eisler, *The Chalice and the Blade: Our History, Our Future* (New York: Harper Collins, 1987).

32. Sherry R. Anderson, *The Feminine Face of God: The Unfolding of the Sacred in Women* (New York, NY: Bantam, 1991).

We were looking for something that would express the feminine rather than the masculine experience of Yoga. We wanted to express the expansive qualities of the feminine, moving to the side and opening. The Sun Salutation is moving in a forward direction, which gives it a goal-oriented expression. We also wanted the poses to be strengthening for women. The goal of the Moon Salutation is to strengthen and open the female anatomy. Therefore, it has a hip-opening series and lateral movements. It is very circular. Menstruation is a part of it, but really it's about all phases of a woman's life. The deep squat is a birthing position and a wonderful position for pregnancy. The slow movements and the hip opening are great for menstruation but good for women in general.

Harriet L. Russell (Bhumi), a senior Kripalu Yoga teacher and co-creator of the Moon Salutation, was especially concerned with the needs of women during menstruation.

I was interested in creating a flow that you could do when you were having your period, that wouldn't have the heaviness of the Sun Salutation. The Moon Salutation works with the female channels. It is softer and flowing, while the Sun Salutation is angular and works with masculine energy. Because it is backwards and forwards, the Sun Salutation heats you more. When you are on your period, you need a flow that is less heating and more cooling.

While the senior female Yoga teachers at Kripalu had spent many years exploring movements that felt good to them and that would be beneficial for their female students, the solidification of these ideas into the actual Moon Salutation took place in a very short time. Deva shared her recollection of the final harnessing of these ideas into a form that could be taught to others:

We knew we wanted to include Crescent Moon Pose and the Goddess Squat, and to combine these with the Full Squat, a powerful birthing pose. When it came to actually writing the flow down, I remember Megha coming into my office and the two of us finalizing it together. Many of us [including Bhumi and Niti] had been experimenting with those postures for years, but it all came together in that one day.

In many ways, the actual generation of this series cannot be attributed to any one group, because these women drew from the collective strength of the ashram as well as the support of the Yoga development team on which they worked. Additionally, many of the poses had originally come from India, while Goddess Pose, or Goddess Squat, had come to Kripalu as a *hara* ("belly" or "center") strengthener from Japan.

The new Moon Salutation was powerfully moving to the students who learned it while on retreat at Kripalu, as well as to its teachers. The staff would dress in white and create a circle facing the program group for their demonstration. Senior Kripalu Yoga teacher and co-creator of the Moon Salutation, Patricia "Niti" Seip Martin, spoke of how eagerly participants received this flow:

We demonstrated the Moon Salutation using spotlights to set the stage for the week and as a centering experience. It was always very powerful for the program group. I think that the power of this experience has been underestimated by many. How do you transmit an experience through seeing? It was always greeted with a great deal of enthusiasm and inspiration by the participants in the class.

The Moon Salutation became a central part of two separate week-long programs: Women and Yoga (first taught in November 1988), and Kripalu Yoga Sadhana Training: Moon Series (first taught in April 1989). While the Moon Salutation had been created specifically for women, the Sadhana Moon Series program was open to women and men, and thus from the very beginning this new flow was taught to all genders.

Patricia remembered how it was taught in these different contexts:

When we did this program exclusively with women we could bring in the physiological aspects of a woman's body and an awareness of the moon. For men, the emphasis is on the belly, a central aspect of the Moon Salutation. For women, the emphasis can be more specifically on the womb.

The Moon Salutation became widely taught at Kripalu. Between 1989 and 1999, both Women and Yoga and the Sadhana Moon Series program were each taught more than 40 times. By 1994, the initial energy that had led to the creation of Women and Yoga began to diversify, and a variety of new programs for women, men, people of color, queer people, youth, and many more emerged. Today, program offerings at Kripalu remain diverse and include a variety of programs specifically for women.

The women who created the Moon Salutation passed it on to new generations of students and teachers after them. The Moon Salutation traveled beyond the walls of Kripalu and out into the world where it continues to grow and to take on a life of its own.

PART TWO: LEARNING MOON SALUTATIONS

8

MEETING THE POSES ~ BODY AND SOUL

Poses are archetypes in the body-mind. We need to uncover them and find a relationship to them.

~ Esther Myers, student of Vanda Scaravelli and
internationally respected Yoga Teacher

This summer, we did the Moon Salutation again around an old oak tree surrounded by a circular stone bench. Our teacher carefully prepared us by teaching one or two poses each day for our first week. Even though I am not practiced in Yoga, I found this tedious, as learning the individual poses felt outer rather than inner ~ and reminded me too much of gym class. But when we were able to do the whole Moon Salutation I was glad for the preparation. The previous summer when I had done it without the preparation, my movements had been awkward, but this time they flowed together.

~ Carol P. Christ, author, *Rebirth of the Goddess: Finding Meaning in Feminine Spirituality*

The Moon Salutation as originally created at Kripalu is formed from nine basic poses, including side bending, forward bending, lunging, and squatting. I call this original sequence the "full circular Moon Salutation," and instructions for putting the poses together in the full flow may be found in Chapter 10.

In this chapter, we'll go steadily through the poses one by one, focusing on their physical and psychological dimensions. Use this chapter to befriend these poses and explore your inner felt sense in each. Also, in this chapter I give options for those with stiff hips, vulnerable knees, or other challenges with range of motion. These modifications will help you adapt the Moon Salutation to keep your body happy, even if you have physical limitations.

If you are a beginner to Yoga, move gently as you start. If at any point you experience pain, stop. Yoga should not hurt! It may be that you need to proceed more slowly or that your body is not meant to do all of the poses. That's fine. You may wish to seek the guidance of an experienced instructor who can show you what is safe for your body. Whatever poses and variations you choose to explore should feel yummy.

Several of the gentle beginning variations shown in Chapter 9 do not require you to learn all of the poses from the full circular Moon Salutation, and you may want to get started with these variations right away. Multiple sequences for beginners and intermediate practitioners are shown in Chapters 9 and 10. You will find ways to expand the flow for increasing challenge in Chapter 11.

If you are already an experienced Yoga practitioner, you may wish to dive right into the full circular Moon Salutation shown in Chapter 10 before reading the psychological dimensions of the individual poses explained here. Be sure you are fully warmed up before attempting the flow your first time. The following chart shows the different variations and modifications to the flow included in this book:

	Learn Quickly in Just a Few Minutes	Accessible to Most Beginners	No deep knee bends or hip opening	Includes deep knee bends and hip opening	Chapter Number
3 Phases of the Moon Flow	●	●	●		9
Moon Salutation with Emphasis on the Belly		●	●		9
Side-to-Side Version		●		(Minimal)	9
Side-to-Side Version with High Lunges	●		●		9
Full Circular Moon Salutation				●	10
Full Circular Moon Salutation with High Lunges			●		10
Breath Modifications	Applicable to any version and all practitioners.				11
Flow Extensions for More Challenge				●	11
Mother Mary Moon Salutation			Can be either		28
Moon Salutation as a Peace Prayer				●	28

Remember that the pose modifications given in this chapter may be used as needed or desired to suit your personal preference or if you have range-of-motion limitations, injury, or pain. Apply these modifications from this chapter to any of the Moon Salutation variations given in Chapters 9 through 11.

The psychological aspects of postures are little known and even less taught. Making this link assumes that the postures activate not only bones and muscles but also psyche and spirit. Swami Sivananda Radha, student of Swami Sivananda of Rishikesh and the founder of Yasodhara Yoga Ashram in Canada, held that the psychological content of posture is found in its actual shape and in the patterns of holding in the bones and muscles.[33]

Transpersonal psychologist Arnold Mindell also maintains that Yoga postures are archetypal in nature, representing potential ways the body may be experienced. Each has a range of possible accompanying moods and symbols that vary according to the context of the practitioner. While the postures emerge spontaneously in different cultures and at different times, Mindell concludes they have been maintained and refined through the centuries due to their archetypal resonance. When students hold the postures and relax the conscious mind, the actual position of the muscles and bones encourages the deeper layer of the posture to emerge. This material is noticed by the observing mind and integrated over time into the deeper psyche.[34]

As we first meet these poses below, we will do the poses to the left side first (for example, we will do Triangle reaching to the left). According to Yogic anatomy, the left side is considered the lunar side of the body, and the right is considered the solar side. In the Moon Salutation, by going to the left side first, we activate the lunar energy and support shifting into the right brain. For some people, it may feel more natural to start with the right side, and it is fine to experiment to discover your preference. However, whichever side you start to, be sure to maintain evenness in the body by practicing the poses to both sides.

---

33. Radha S. Saraswati, *Hatha Yoga: The Hidden Language: Symbols, Secrets, and Metaphor* (*Spokane, WA: Timeless Books,* 1995) integrates discussion of the physical aspects of the postures with their symbolic and mythological content.

34. Arnold Mindell. *Dreambody: The Body's Role in Revealing the Self* (Boston: Sigo Press, 1982).

1. Mountain Pose

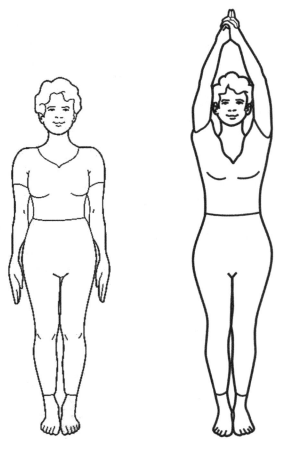

Mountain Pose

Temple Pose
(Variation of Mountain)[35]

Entering the Pose

The Moon Salutation begins with Mountain Pose. Stand with your feet rooted firmly on the earth, big toes touching, and the crown of the head reaching up to the sky. The entire body stretches between these two poles. Feel the movement of the breath conducting energy from earth to sky.

---

35. Photo model this chapter the author, some photos from 1998, some from 2019.

After taking a few breaths here to ground into your body, sweep the arms out to the side on an inhalation, and bring them overhead. Relax the shoulders down and away from the ears. Interlace the fingers overhead with index fingers extended. This variation of Mountain Pose with arms overhead is called Temple Pose.

Options

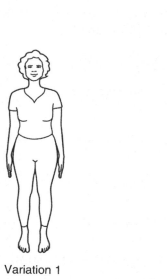 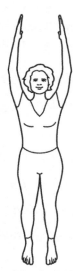

Variation 1   Variation 2

If it is uncomfortable or difficult to balance with the feet touching in this pose, place the feet hip-width distance apart (var. 1). When the arms are overhead, you can keep the arms separated rather than bringing hands together (var. 2). This may be helpful for those with tight shoulders or pain in the shoulders.

Benefits

Physically, Mountain is strengthening and steadying. It strengthens the muscles of the feet and legs, developing and protecting the arches of the feet, the ankles, and the knee joints. Strong legs in turn provide a healthy foundation for the rest of the body. Stretching the torso upward and rolling the shoulders back help to counteract the forward slump and rounded spine so often found in our culture as a result of sedentary lifestyle, poor posture, and the overwhelming prevalence of mobile phones and laptops. A lifted posture gives room to the heart and lungs so that they may function optimally.

Experiencing the Pose

Psychologically, Mountain invites a calm exploration of one's own nature. The neutral and open position of the torso allows one to go deeply within while also feeling connected to the cosmos without. Swami Radha says that reflections such as the following may arise while practicing Mountain Pose:

standing still, not running somewhere;

standing still, looking - without, within;

standing still, taking stock;

standing still, observing . . .

standing still, feeling . . .

standing still, seeing . . .

standing still, asking: Where am I?[36]

As the arms open to the sides in preparation for Temple Pose, there is a sense of reaching out and opening to all life. In Temple Pose itself, there is also a conscious awareness of needing to open the heart. Further, having the arms overhead creates an active sense of engaging with life as opposed to the more passive experience of arms by the sides.

---

36. Radha S. Saraswati, *Hatha Yoga, 32* (Italics and ellipsis in the original).

2. CRESCENT MOON POSE

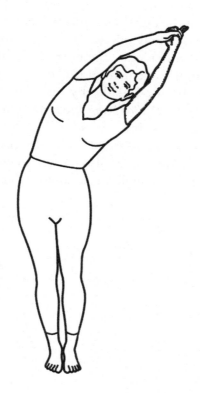

Entering the Pose

From Temple, the body moves into the shape of the crescent moon. To come into Crescent Moon Pose, lift up through the ribs and waist, lift the pelvic floor, gently squeeze the buttocks, and bend the upper body slightly to the left while the hips move slightly to the right. Keep the heart open, facing forward, and the body long. If you feel any strain in the lower back, bend less, returning closer to upright.

   * Note: As mentioned above, we are beginning these poses to the left side, and you can imagine that you are embodying the model. If you would prefer to begin to the right, simply reverse the written instructions.

Options

In the Moon Salutation, entering this pose may be synchronized with the rhythm of the breath; the practitioner might exhale while softening to the side and inhale while reaching upward again, then repeat to the other side. The flow of the breath in this way supports the natural movement of the torso. In my experience, it also creates a steady side-to-side rhythm that is similar in effect to the practice of *nadi shodhana* (alternate nostril breathing), considered to be balancing and soothing. Some practitioners prefer to move more slowly and to hold Crescent Moon Pose for several breaths. You might also choose to enter the pose very slowly, inching into it a little more with each breath, extending and lengthening the body as you go.

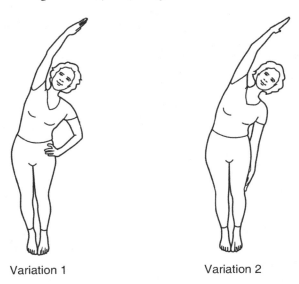

Variation 1   Variation 2

If the back is uncomfortable or feels strained as you bend to one side, or if there is sacroiliac pain, place one hand on the hip as you bend towards that side for more support (var. 1). Another option is to let that hand slide down the leg (var. 2). Do not bend as deeply.

Benefits

Crescent Moon strengthens and stretches the large muscles of the torso, particularly the side-bending muscles. It also tones the legs, hips, and arms, creates space between the ribs, and releases adhesions from between the ribs that can prevent a full and easy breath. This in turn prevents the gradual calcification of the joints between the ribs and sternum and the ribs and spine, maintaining the freedom to breathe fully as one ages. Bending the torso in this way also massages the internal organs, providing a fresh supply of blood after completion of the posture. For this reason Crescent Moon is considered to benefit the liver, spleen, kidneys, and digestive organs.

Experiencing the Pose

Bending in and out of Crescent Moon creates a sense of self that changes comfortably with the flux of nature rather than needing to control it. Its rhythm evokes other rhythms - the tides, lunar cycle, waves on a beach, the flow of emotions and feelings, the monthly menstrual cycle. The openness in the heart joined with the flow of this motion creates a sense of soft courage, openness, compassion, and wisdom.

Particularly while flowing in and out of Crescent Moon, I feel myself to be a moon goddess. I have often resisted the expression of my own softness, preferring to protect myself from being dismissed as "feminine" by being strong and forceful. Practicing Crescent Moon Pose invites me to accept the softer, flowing parts of myself and to recognize their beauty.

3. GODDESS POSE

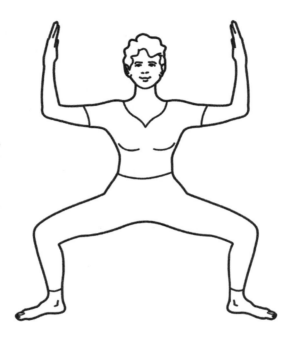

Entering the Pose

To enter Goddess Pose, step the left foot to the side and bend both knees, coming into a wide squat. Bend the elbows at left angles so the palms face each other. Use the inner thigh muscles to open the thighs wide, deepening the squat. The kneecaps should be pointed in the same direction as the toes to protect the knees and ankles. Feel the pelvis being supported by the strength of the thighs, and feel the root chakra, the *muladhara*, being deeply opened.

Options

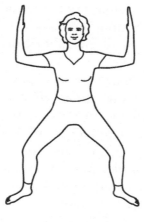

Variation 1

If the knees feel any pain, try bending them less deeply.

Benefits

Goddess Pose is both grounding and releasing. It strengthens the arm muscles as well as the leg muscles, particularly the thighs but also the hips, knees, and feet. It stretches the hips and groin wide, bringing blood and circulation to the inner thighs and pelvic region. Dropping deeply into Goddess Pose requires both flexibility in the hips and strength in the core (inner torso muscles); these are developed with practice.

Experiencing the Pose

Originally known as Victory Squat, this pose has come to be known as Goddess Pose due to the way it is felt by many to be "such a strong female stance."[37] I love to call it "Lioness," and I've also heard it called "Kali Pose." This position is found cross-culturally in sacred art, both as a birthing posture and in contexts of *yoni* worship (where the female genitals and birth canal

---

37. Deva Parnell, personal interview with author, June 21, 1999.

are revered).[38] Opening the hips wide with knees bent creates a deep opening not only in the body but also in the psyche. For many people this pose is likely to evoke feelings of deep connection to the earth, of owning one's sexuality, of celebrating one's power, and of awareness of metaphoric or actual connection to giving birth.

Yoga innovator Arthur Kilmurray says that this pose evokes deep memory of one's pre-verbal self. He places it, along with other groin stretches, in the category of Frog Pose.[39] Many women speak of entering their "reptilian brain" during labor, of losing all track of time and entering a deeper, older part of their psyche. Perhaps these poses of physical openness in the belly and groin activate the ancient memory in both men and women of a time before the evolution of conscious thought. They are a return to the primitive world of feeling, sexuality, sensuality, and birth.

Some students find that squatting with the knees wide open creates a sense of honoring the womb. Kripalu Yoga teacher Lisa Sarasohn lists this pose as one of those that focus awareness on the belly.[40] Called the *hara* in Japanese, the belly is considered sacred in Eastern cultures; many meditational movement practices aim at gathering energy in this region. This pose was originally brought to Kripalu as a hara-, or belly-strengthener.

For me, this pose also evokes a centered fierceness, a sense of protecting the earth, nature, and those more vulnerable than I. A student of mine once reflected on her sense that the pose's strength is feminine in nature, saying that it "is strong, but in a way that is completely free of testosterone. It's more of a steady than an aggressive strength." This pose is powerful in the way that a lioness protects her child. Here is the energy of Kali, the fierce warrior goddess who is also a compassionate mother.

---

38. For examples in tantrism, see Ajit Mookerjee and Madhu Khanna, *The Tantric Way: Art, Science, Ritual* (London: Thames & Hudson, 1977) and Ajit Mookerjee, *Kali: The Feminine Force* (Rochester, NY: Destiny Books, 1988).

39. Arthur Kilmurray, "Yoga for Hips and Thighs," *Yoga Journal* 90 (May/June 1989).

40. Lisa Sarasohn, "Honoring the Belly," *Yoga Journal* 121 (July/August 1993).

4. FIVE-POINTED STAR POSE

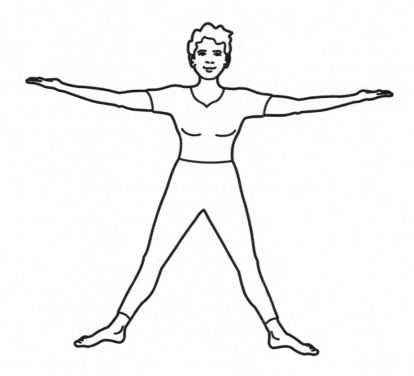

Entering the Pose

To come into Five-Pointed Star Pose, straighten the legs and extend the arms to the sides, palms facing up. Relax the shoulders away from the ears and open the chest wide. Engage the leg muscles, drawing them up and away from the floor.

Options

Turn the palms to face down (not pictured).

Benefits

Physically, this pose strengthens the legs, torso, and arms as the body is extended as widely as possible in all directions. Slow inhalation while the arms and legs reach outwards invites a deep breath naturally into the lungs.

Experiencing the Pose

Psychologically, there is a feeling of joy in extending the arms and legs, of celebrating one's existence. There is spaciousness and a sense of freeing one's spirit outward. In some ways this pose is similar to Mountain, the first pose in the series. Yet Mountain, with arms neutrally by the sides, is more a simple statement and contemplation of one's nature. This pose, with arms and legs spread wide, celebrates that nature.

According to John Willey, Director of Yoga Teacher Training at Kripalu Center in the 1990s, the energy channels that run from hands to heart and from feet to navel are energized as they lengthen in this pose; the solar plexus is the bridge between the two. This expansion of the energy channels contributes to the sense of vitality experienced in Five-Pointed Star.

The shape of Five-Pointed Star is found in art as an expression and/or celebration of quintessential humanness. An example is the famous sketch by Leonardo da Vinci that shows the proportions of a man's limbs. The subject stands with arms and legs outstretched, creating reverberations of beauty and form. This pose is an archetypal expression of joy in our sacred geometry.

Energetically, this joy extends from the physical body outward to the wider universe. I have experienced this in different ways – as energy spiraling out from my body into the universe, as energy entering me from without through my arms and legs, or as the body acting as a conduit of this energy. The pulsation of creation is strongly felt. Five-Pointed Star Pose is a way of gathering energy from heaven and earth and storing it in the belly.[41]

---

41. Sarasohn, "Honoring the Belly," *Yoga Journal* 121 (July/August 1993).

5. Triangle Pose

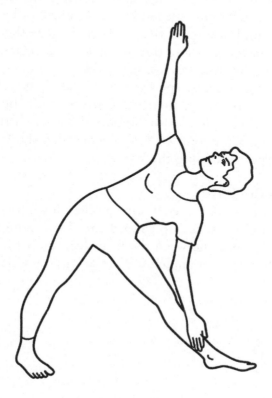

Preparing for the Pose

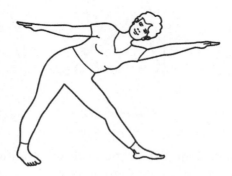

Prepare for Triangle from Five-Pointed Star by first turning the left foot out to the side and turning in the right foot so it points straight ahead. Turn out the left thigh using the hip and thigh muscles, and make sure the left kneecap points in the same direction as the middle toes of the left foot. Engage the leg muscles and reach the left arm and the entire torso to the left, stretching through the ribs as far as is comfortable.

Be careful not to hyperextend the left knee which would press back into the ligaments and overstretch them. Instead, engage the thigh muscles to support the knee, lifting through the kneecap. Bend your left knee ever so slightly if you need to prevent hyper-extending the knee.

Entering the Pose

Shift the arms so that the left arm reaches down toward the shin while the right reaches up toward the sky. Rotate the head to look up. The space between the front leg, lower ribs, and lower arm should form a triangle, just as the legs do with the floor.

Options

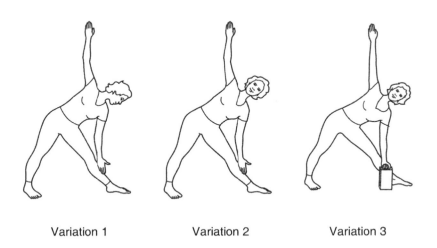

Variation 1   Variation 2   Variation 3

If there is any discomfort in the neck or shoulders, look down or straight ahead with neck aligned with the spine (var. 1 or var. 2). A block may also be placed under the left fingertips or hand, providing additional support to lengthen the body (var. 3).

Benefits

This pose strengthens the feet, legs, and hips, particularly working the muscles that support and turn out the thighs. It opens and stretches the groin and inner thighs. It gently twists the back, relieving lower back pain. It creates opening in the ribs and across the chest.

Experiencing the Pose

Psychologically, this pose is a combination of stability and suppleness, stability being found in the triangle shape of the legs and suppleness in the reach of the upper body. As with Crescent Moon, enter Triangle by reaching gracefully to the side. This creates the sense of inner flexibility and a willingness to flow with the cycles and elements of nature.

According to Swami Radha, the triangle is both the most stable figure in construction and a spiritually potent symbol; it represents the unity of body, mind, and spirit. She says, "When physical balance has been achieved in the practice of this asana, a sharper picture will emerge of the balance required in all areas of life."[42]

While holding this pose, we are also able to reflect on the guidance we receive from universal spirit and how we might wish to make better use of that guidance.

---

42. Radha S. Saraswati, *Hatha Yoga*.

6. Pyramid Pose

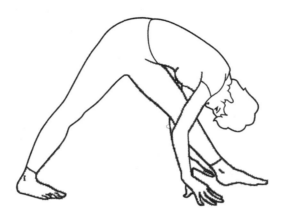

Entering the Pose

To come into this position from Triangle Pose, circle the upper arm over toward the ear and then down toward the floor. Place one hand on either side of the left foot and adjust the hips so that they evenly face the left leg. You may need to shorten your stance somewhat, bringing the right leg in closer to the left, so that you can square the hips. If the hamstrings are very tight, the front knee may bend slightly. Both feet are flat on the ground; adjust the back foot if you need to so that it stays flat. Press down into the heel of the back foot and the ball of the front foot. Relax the neck completely.

Options

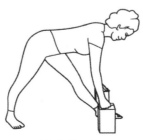

Variation 1

If your leg muscles are tight so that it is difficult to reach the floor, or if there is any back pain, try putting a block on either side of the front foot on which to place your hands.

Benefits

This pose strengthens the legs, stretches the hamstring and back muscles, and gives a gentle massage to the abdominal organs. Because the legs are spread wide, this pose is one of the few forward bends that may be safely practiced during pregnancy; there is room for the belly to the side of the front leg.

Experiencing the Pose

Forward bends represent humility and a drawing into oneself. The practitioner enjoys a sense of release and inner quiet. This pose is also a gentle inversion, bringing fresh blood to the head and fresh ideas to the mind. Turning one's view of the world upside down in this way can evoke new perspective on aspects of your life that have become habitual.

7. LUNGE POSE

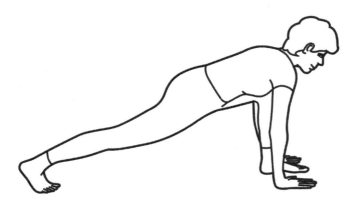

Entering the Pose

In Lunge Pose, the front knee bends at ninety degrees while the other leg stretches back. Reach the back foot far enough behind that the front knee is aligned directly above the front ankle. Relax the shoulders and neck as you gently gaze forward. Lower the hips as far as is comfortable without bending the back knee.

Options

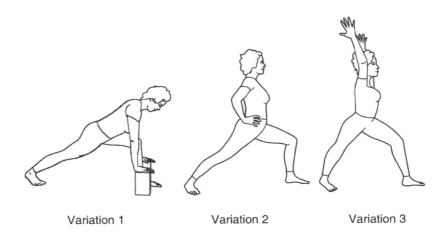

Variation 1   Variation 2   Variation 3

If it is hard to reach the ground or if there is pain in Lunge Pose, try placing a block on either side of the front foot on which to put your hands (var. 1). Or if the hips and knees are more comfortable, come a little bit higher into Warrior One Pose, either with hands on hips (var. 2) or hands by the ears (var. 3). In any of these options, the left knee remains bent and forward, the right leg is back and straight, and the torso faces the front knee.

Benefits

This pose gives a deep stretch across the groin, also stretching the hip, thigh, and calf. It is also a very gentle backbend that massages the kidneys and adrenal glands. Lunge Pose creates a feeling of reaching out to the future, of preparing to take action, of motion.[43] As the heart opens forward in the gentle backbend, there is a sense of courage and openness.

Experiencing the Pose

In Sanskrit, Lunge Pose is named after Anjani, mother of the monkey god Hanuman. Hanuman is the patron saint of those who practice *seva* (selfless service). This pose honors the readiness to serve and the feminine principle that gives birth to such readiness. The pose embodies humility, because one is low to the ground; courage, because of the open heart; and a willingness to serve, because of the sense of stepping forward.[44] The same qualities may be felt in Warrior One Pose.

In the Moon Salutation, Lunge serves as a transition from the standing, or upper-world poses to the lower down, fully squatting, low-to-the-ground poses. Thus, this descent occurs within the context of humility and courage.

I also experience the pose as a prayer for protection and a request for grace as I continue on my journey. Megha Nancy Buttenheim, one of the co-creators of the Moon Salutation, refers to this sense of blessings on her audiotape *Beyond Limits: Moon Series*, in which she suggests that the practitioner in this pose look up to receive a "moon bath."[45] In this pose one receives blessings from the divine world above in preparation for the journey ahead.

---

43. It is also part of the Sun Salutation, where it similarly carries the sense of motion into the future.

44. John Friend, "*Anjaneyasana*," *Yoga Journal* 142 (September/October 1998).

45. Nancy Megha Buttenheim, *Beyond Limits: Moon Series* (Lenox, MA: Kripalu Center, 1991).

8. SIDE LUNGE POSE

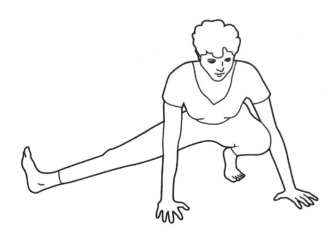

Entering the Pose

To enter Side Lunge from Lunge, the hips and torso rotate ninety degrees to face forward and the flexed right foot shifts onto its heel, toes pointing up. The legs and hips stay low to the ground and the left knee stays bent while the right leg stays long. Bring both hands forward and the weight forward so that the hips are over the ball of the left foot. Engage the muscles of the right thigh to prevent hyperextension of the knee.

    * Note: this can be a challenging pose for many people. If your hips are tight or if you have ever had knee pain, I recommend substituting Warrior Two Pose shown in the options below.

    Also, if you are very flexible, you may be able to lower the heel of the squatting leg to the floor. But be careful not to over-stretch the ligaments under the knee of the straight leg. Flexing the foot of the extended leg will help to engage the quadriceps muscle and add protection to the knee.

Options

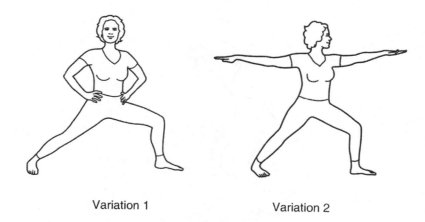

Variation 1   Variation 2

If you have tight hips or vulnerable knees, use Warrior Two instead of Side Lunge Pose, providing you a gentler way to experience the Moon Salutation. Hands may be on hips (var. 1) or extended to the side (var. 2), head facing forward or to the side as you prefer.

Benefits

Side Lunge or Warrior Two offer a deep opening to the inner thighs and pelvis. This pose is considered highly beneficial for women because of the stretch across the uterus and ovaries, similar to either Seated or Standing Wide-Legged Stretch.[46]

Experiencing the Pose

When in the full Side Lunge, I prefer to teach this pose with the upper body softening forward on the exhalation. For me, softening the upper body toward the ground enhances connection with the earth, and I feel in this connection a deep honoring of nature; I experience her in these moments as blessed Mother. Often, this pose brings up intimate memories of the earth ~ cornfields and ponds near my childhood home, a special hiding place where I would receive wisdom, and later touching the earth in sorrow as I became aware of the damage being done to her by human hands. Perhaps it is the soft touch of my hands on the ground that stirs these memories.

---

46. Geeta S. Iyengar, *Yoga: A Gem for Women* (Spokane, WA: Timeless Books, 1990).

9. Full Squat Pose

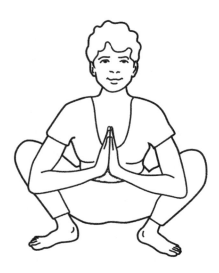

Entering the Pose

The Full Squat is the central pose of the full circular Moon
Salutation. Some call this Birthing Pose or Frog Pose. In this
pose, the knees bend deeply and the hips drop down toward the
ground. The elbows are placed inside the knees, opening them
outward. The palms touch each other in front of the heart.

* Note: Very flexible practitioners may find that their heels
come flat on the ground. In order to prevent straining the knees
or ankles, the knees should be pointing in the same direction
as the toes. It is important not to sacrifice the integrity of these
joints in order to force the heels down before the body is ready.
While lowering the heels is satisfying and grounding, it is certainly not necessary.

Options

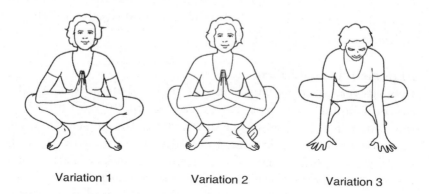

Variation 1   Variation 2   Variation 3

If the heels do not touch the ground, try to widen the stance (var. 1), or place a folded blanket under the heels (var. 2). If balance is difficult with the heels up and no blanket is available, the hands may stay on the floor (var. 3).

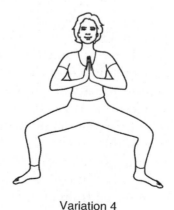

Variation 4

If the knees do not want to bend so deeply, return to Goddess Pose (var. 4) with hands at the heart. Goddess Pose also flows well from Warrior One and Warrior Two Poses if you are using those variations to Lunge and Side Lunge.

Benefits

Physically, Full Squat encourages relaxation and openness in the groin. It releases the muscles of the lower buttocks and spine, easing lower-back pain.

Experiencing the Pose

In whatever variation, this is an extremely earthy pose. Literally, the Full Squat is as close as one can get to the ground while remaining in the active stance of standing. The most vulnerable part of the body is wide open and left next to the earth. As with Goddess Pose, Full Squat is found frequently in sacred art, where it celebrates a powerful femininity. In pre-modern cultures, it is a quintessential posture for childbirth. While in modern cultures, women may be strapped on their backs during labor, ancient cultures preferred the squatting posture, giving women dignity and strength and allowing gravity to help with the birth. This is also the posture of other sorts of laborers. Men and women often assume this low squat as they work in the fields or sell their wares.

On an even more basic level, the Full Squat was the posture of defecating before the advent of flush (or "Western") toilets. While many of us feel shame at human body functions, in the Moon Salutation we are reminded of the sanctity of all things. Our intimate connection to earth is found in the nourishing processes of eating, digestion, and excretion, as well as in the creative processes of sexuality and childbirth. All of these connections are contained in this pose.

In our Western culture, we have completely lost contact with this posture. It is foreign and uncomfortable for many of us. Similarly, we are disconnected from our place in the web of life, and so live in ways that daily weaken our life-support structures. Learning to "hang out" (literally and figuratively) in this pose may be one of the ways back to our connection to the planet.

9
GENTLE BEGINNER MOON SALUTATIONS

I find the Moon Salutation much more accessible than the Sun Salutation. People with a wider range of (non) abilities ~ those with limited flexibility ~ are more easily able to engage in it than the Sun Salute.

~ Valerie Renwick, Yoga Instructor

A good jumping-off point for total beginners is the Three Phases of the Moon Flow shown below. As you gain familiarity with more of the poses from the previous chapter, go on to explore the Gentle Moon Salutation with Emphasis on the Belly. Then try one of the Side-to-Side Variations given next in this chapter. These beginner sequences allow you to link most of the poses from the full circular Moon Salutation while omitting some of the trickier transitions that can be tough for newcomers. Choose from either the "high lunge" version if your hips are tight (Variation 4 below) or the "low lunge" version for more flexible bodies (Variation 3 below). Enjoy!

1. THREE PHASES OF THE MOON FLOW

This flow will give you the feel of the contrast between the open-hearted side-bending postures of Crescent Moon Pose and the inward quiet of Dark Moon Pose (a modified forward bend). It can be practiced standing or seated on a chair or side of the bed, making it highly accessible either as a pre-bedtime ritual or as a sequence for those with special needs. This is also a wonderful variation for large groups, who learn it quickly and easily, and then readily tune in to the flow of breath with movement. [47]

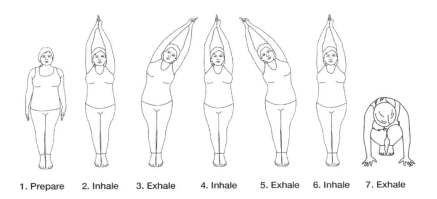

1. Prepare   2. Inhale   3. Exhale   4. Inhale   5. Exhale   6. Inhale   7. Exhale

Three Phases of the Moon Flow Steps

1. Mountain Pose, hands by sides.
2. Inhale, trace the shape of the Full Moon with the hands and bring the arms overhead to Temple (interlace fingers, extend index fingers).
3. Exhale, Crescent Moon left. [48]
4. Inhale, Temple.
5. Exhale, Crescent Moon right.
6. Inhale, Temple.
7. Exhale, Dark Moon (knees bend fully, body rounds down over knees, head is down, hands touch the ground, or for more challenge, hands wrap around shins).
8. Pause for three full breaths in Dark Moon.
9. Repeat from Step 2 above.

---

47. Photo model Maria Arvayo.

48. As described in Chapter 8, we are beginning all flows to the left side. To follow the pictures imagine that you are embodying the model. If you would prefer to begin to the right, simply reverse the written instructions.

10. Continue for as many repetitions as desired.

11. When ready to complete, inhale, Temple, and then exhale, arms to sides to Mountain.

I like to teach this flow by giving the instructions verbally, continuing for several rounds, and then concluding with a silent round in which the group stays together by listening to others' breathing. Those with knee trouble in squatting can simply come into a gentle forward bend in Dark Moon Pose (#7 above) instead of coming into a deep knee bend.

2. GENTLE MOON SALUTATION WITH EMPHASIS ON THE BELLY

Similar to the previous variation, this flow is also appropriate for large groups, including large groups of beginners.[49] It omits any deep knee bends and includes a gentle version of Triangle. It includes Five-Pointed Star, Goddess and a modified Triangle Pose, while omitting the Lunges, Pyramid Pose, and Full Squat. It is thus easier on hips and knees. It adds Wide-Legged Forward Bend and Twisting Wide-Legged Forward Bend, two new poses. If the hamstrings are tight, put a block in front of you on which to place your hands during Wide-Legged Forward Bend Pose.

This variation also brings the hands to the belly, emphasizing the womb-like elements of the flow. I find the movement with the breath out of Crescent Moon back to hands at the belly very quieting and centering. Going into Five-Pointed Star from the hands-on-belly position also helps to emphasize the belly aspects of Five-Pointed Star and Goddess Poses.[50]

---

49. This variation was first shared with me by Sudha Carolyn Lundeen, RN, Yoga teacher trainer.

50. Photo model Denise Alston.

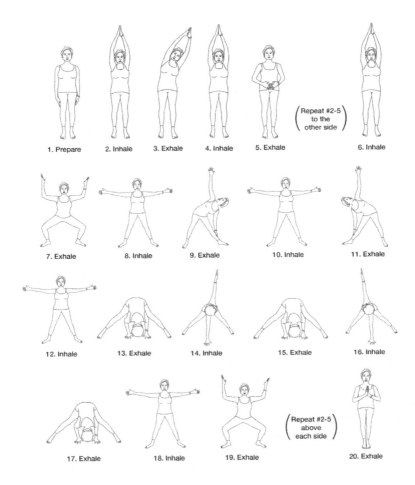

1. Prepare   2. Inhale   3. Exhale   4. Inhale   5. Exhale   6. Inhale

7. Exhale   8. Inhale   9. Exhale   10. Inhale   11. Exhale

12. Inhale   13. Exhale   14. Inhale   15. Exhale   16. Inhale

17. Exhale   18. Inhale   19. Exhale   20. Exhale

Gentle Moon Salutation with Emphasis on the Belly Steps

1. Begin in Mountain.
2. Inhale, sweep arms out to sides and overhead to Temple.
3. Exhale, Crescent Moon left.
4. Inhale, Temple.
5. Exhale, arms sweep out to sides, hands come to rest over belly.

Repeat Steps 2–5 above for Crescent Moon to the right.

6. Inhale, arms up to Temple.
7. Exhale, Goddess.
8. Inhale, Five-Pointed Star.
9. Exhale, Triangle left (left hand glides down leg toward left calf).
10. Inhale, Five-Pointed Star.
11. Exhale, Triangle right.
12. Inhale, Five-Pointed Star.
13. Exhale, Wide-Legged Forward Bend (hands on floor or block directly below shoulders).
14. Inhale, Twisting Wide-Legged Forward Bend left (left arm raises up towards ceiling, eyes on fingers).
15. Exhale, Wide-Legged Forward Bend.
16. Inhale, Twisting Wide-Legged Forward Bend right.
17. Exhale, Wide-Legged Forward Bend.
18. Inhale, 5-Pointed Star (bend knees and roll up to standing).
19. Exhale, Goddess.

Repeat Steps 2-5 above, each side.

20. Exhale, arms come down to the side, tracing the shape of the Full Moon.

Repeat to the other side. Moving slowly with attention on breath and detail draws the attention inward. Moving rapidly creates a more aerobic flow.

3. SIDE-TO-SIDE MOON SALUTATION

Here you will flow through Five-Pointed Star, Triangle, Pyramid Pose, and Lunge Poses to one side of the body and then return to Goddess, continuing the flow to the other side of the body. This variation omits Side Lunge and Full Squat, two poses that can be tough for beginners or for those with tight hips or vulnerable knees. It also omits the subtle transitions that can be confusing for the uninitiated, such as entering Triangle from below in Pyramid Pose or the transitions from Lunge to Side Lunge and the reverse on the other leg.[51]

---

51. Photo model Reed Kolber.

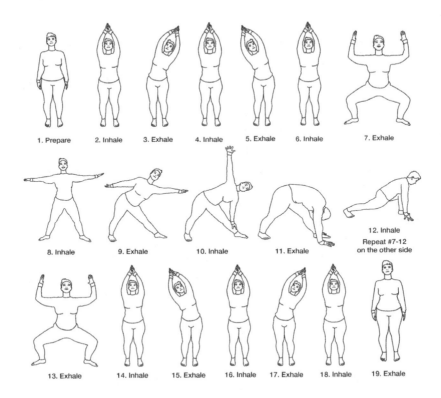

1. Prepare   2. Inhale   3. Exhale   4. Inhale   5. Exhale   6. Inhale   7. Exhale

8. Inhale   9. Exhale   10. Inhale   11. Exhale   12. Inhale
Repeat #7-12
on the other side

13. Exhale   14. Inhale   15. Exhale   16. Inhale   17. Exhale   18. Inhale   19. Exhale

Side-to-Side Moon Salutation Steps

1. Begin in Mountain with hands by sides.
2. Inhale, sweep arms out to sides and overhead to Temple (interlace fingers, extend index fingers).
3. Exhale, Crescent Moon left.
4. Inhale, Temple.
5. Exhale, Crescent Moon right.
6. Inhale, Temple.
7. Exhale, Goddess.
8. Inhale, Five-Pointed Star.
9. Exhale, Triangle preparation left (left foot turns out, right foot slightly in, torso reaches left with head in line with spine, arms reach left staying parallel to floor).
10. Inhale, Triangle left (arms rotate with left arm pointing to floor, right arm to ceiling).

11. Exhale, Pyramid Pose (sweep right arm by ear and to floor, rotate hips to face left).
12. Inhale, Lunge.

Repeat Steps 7 - 12 above to the right.

13. Exhale, Goddess.
14. Inhale, Temple.
15. Exhale, Crescent Moon right.
16. Inhale, Temple.
17. Exhale, Crescent Moon left.
18. Inhale, Temple.
19. Sweep arms to sides slowly through the shape of the Full Moon, taking several breaths if desired.
20. Repeat to the other side.

4. Side-to-Side Moon Salutation with High Lunges

This is a somewhat gentler version of the sequence above, omitting Lunge Pose, which can be difficult to reach for some, and instead substituting Warrior One and Warrior Two Poses. Warrior Two eases the transition into Goddess before going to the second side, while Warrior One is more accessible to those for whom the lower-to-the-ground Lunge Pose is difficult.[52]

---

52. Photo model Anh Chi Pham.

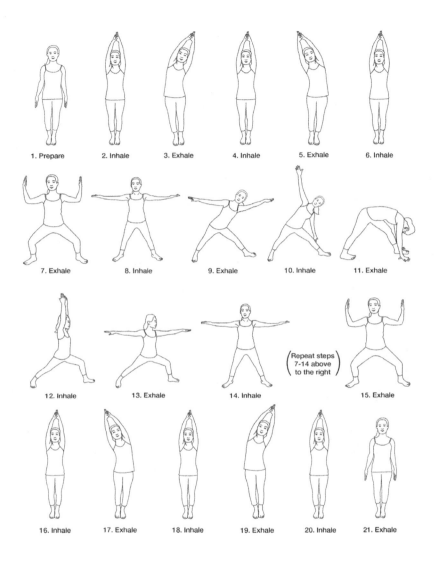

Moon Salutation Side-to-Side Variation with High Lunges Steps

1. Begin in Mountain with hands by sides.
2. Inhale, sweep arms out to sides and overhead to Temple (interlace fingers, extend index fingers).
3. Exhale, Crescent Moon left.
4. Inhale, Temple.

5. Exhale, Crescent Moon right.
6. Inhale, Temple.
7. Exhale, Goddess.
8. Inhale, Five-Pointed Star.
9. Exhale, Triangle preparation left (left foot turns out, right foot slightly in, torso reaches left with head in line with spine, arms reach left staying parallel to floor).
10. Inhale, Triangle left (arms rotate with left arm pointing to floor, right arm to ceiling).
11. Exhale, Pyramid Pose (sweep right arm by ear and to floor, rotate hips to face left).
12. Inhale, Warrior One.
13. Exhale, Warrior Two.
14. Inhale, Star

Repeat Steps 7 - 14 above to the right.

15. Exhale, Goddess.
16. Inhale, Temple.
17. Exhale, Crescent Moon right.
18. Inhale, Temple.
19. Exhale, Crescent Moon left.
20. Inhale, Temple.
21. Sweep arms to sides slowly through the shape of the Full Moon, taking several breaths if desired.
22. Repeat to the other side.

10

FULL CIRCULAR MOON SALUTATIONS

*Doing the Moon Salutation one time through felt like the
perfect amount of exercise to wake me up and soften my body.
We had been urged by our teacher to modify the poses to suit
our bodies. I did not force myself to come all the way down in
Pyramid Pose or the second squat. I like the sequence of the poses:
softening, opening, reaching, bending, squatting. The squat
makes me feel especially strong and female and connected to
something very ancient.*

~ Carol P. Christ, author, *Rebirth of the Goddess: Finding
Meaning in Feminine Spirituality*

In this chapter, we will explore the full circular Moon Salutation
as first created at Kripalu. This chapter gives two ways to
practice a circular Moon Salutation, either with low lunges
(the original version first created at Kripalu, shown in the graphic
above) or with high lunges (shown in a later section of this chapter). The high lunge version is more accessible for those with stiff
hips or knees, or for anyone who simply wishes to avoid deep
knee bends.

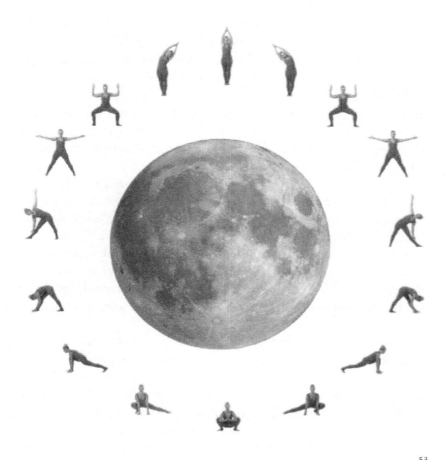

53

Sequencing the poses in the form of a circle ~ whether with high or low lunges ~ creates a sense of wholeness and completeness. It puts practitioners in a dreamy state, the more exploratory, open space of *eros*. Moving into this lunar mode of being is an important aspect of the Moon Salutation; it is what complements the Sun Salutation so well. Those whose bodies are better served by omitting low lunges can still enjoy the circularity and flow of the complete Moon Salutation simply by making a few pose substitutions as shown below.

At the same time, the classic Moon Salutation with low lunges has several features that strengthen how well it complements

53. Photo Credit David Lurey, Find Balance Yoga. Model Mirjam Wagner.

the Sun Salutation. It includes all the phases of the moon ~ the darkness of the new moon (in the lower-to-the-ground poses such as Side Lunge and Full Squat) as well as the radiance of the full moon (Five-Pointed Star, the arm movement from Temple to hands in front of the heart at the close). This honors the dark and light inherent in all of our lives and in women's life cycles in particular. The full Moon Salutation in this way enacts the mysteries of death and rebirth, something I'll explore further in Chapter 23.

Further, the classic flow with low lunges includes the Full Squat as centerpiece. Full Squat is a wonderful counterbalance to Cobra, the centerpiece of the Sun Salutation. Cobra is the primary pose for raising the body's energy, while Full Squat unequivocally grounds that energy, bringing us back to valuing our connection to the earth and to truly honoring our embodiment. For all of these reasons, the full Moon Salutation has a psychological and spiritual power for both women and men that meets and balances that of the Sun Salutation.

One note of caution: Some people believe they have injured their knees from practicing the full circular Moon Salutation with low lunges repeatedly. I personally believe that Side Lunge can be hard on knees, even if practiced correctly. For this reason, I decided not to practice this variation on a daily basis over an extended period. Instead, I save the flow for special occasions, such as when demonstrating in a workshop or in my personal practice for three days each on new or full moons.

FULL CIRCULAR MOON SALUTATION STEPS[54]

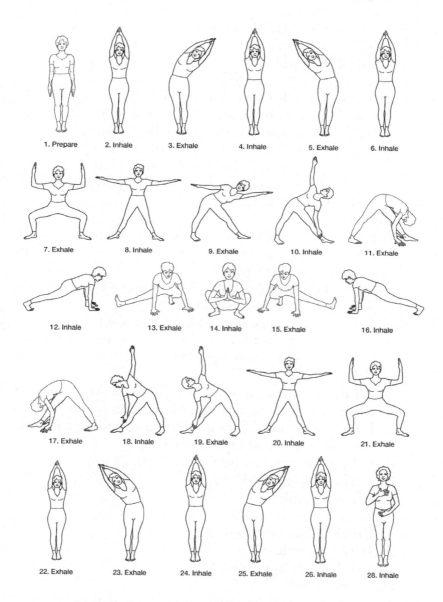

1. Prepare   2. Inhale   3. Exhale   4. Inhale   5. Exhale   6. Inhale

7. Exhale   8. Inhale   9. Exhale   10. Inhale   11. Exhale

12. Inhale   13. Exhale   14. Inhale   15. Exhale   16. Inhale

17. Exhale   18. Inhale   19. Exhale   20. Inhale   21. Exhale

22. Exhale   23. Exhale   24. Inhale   25. Exhale   26. Inhale   28. Inhale

1. Begin in Mountain with hands by sides.
2. Inhale, sweep arms out to sides and overhead to Temple (interlace fingers, extend first fingers and thumbs).

---

54. Photo model the author.

3. Exhale, Crescent Moon left.[55]
4. Inhale, Temple.
5. Exhale, Crescent Moon right.
6. Inhale, Temple.
7. Exhale, Goddess.
8. Inhale, Five-Pointed Star.
9. Exhale, Triangle preparation left (left foot turns out, right foot slightly in, torso reaches left with head in line with spine, arms reach left staying parallel to floor).
10. Inhale, Triangle left (arms shift with left arm pointing to floor, right arm to ceiling, turn head to look up).
11. Exhale, Pyramid Pose (sweep right arm by ear and to floor, rotate hips to face left).
12. Inhale, Lunge.
13. Exhale, Side Lunge (walk hands front, rotate hips to face forward bringing weight over left toes, see options in Chapter 8 or 9 if needed).
14. Inhale, Full Squat (see options in Chapter 8 or 9 if needed). Take three complete breaths.
15. Exhale, Side Lunge (extend left leg to side).
16. Inhale, Lunge (walk hands over to the right – one on either side of the bent right knee).
17. Exhale, Pyramid.
18. Inhale, Triangle preparation right (eyes stay down for balance, prepare feet with right foot out, left in slightly, bring both arms in front of right knee, open left arm up, open shoulders and hips into Triangle).
19. Exhale, Triangle (rotate the head to look up).
20. Inhale, Five-Pointed Star.
21. Exhale, Goddess.
22. Inhale, Temple.
23. Exhale, Crescent Moon right.
24. Inhale, Temple.
25. Exhale, Crescent Moon left.
26. Inhale, Temple.
27. Sweep arms to sides slowly through the shape of the Full Moon, taking several breaths if desired.

---

55. Again, as described in Chapter 8, we are beginning all flows to the left side. To follow the pictures imagine that you are embodying the model. If you would prefer to begin to the right, simply reverse the written instructions.

28. Rest with one hand on belly, one hand on heart.
29. Repeat to the other side.

FULL CIRCULAR MOON SALUTATION WITH HIGH LUNGES[56]

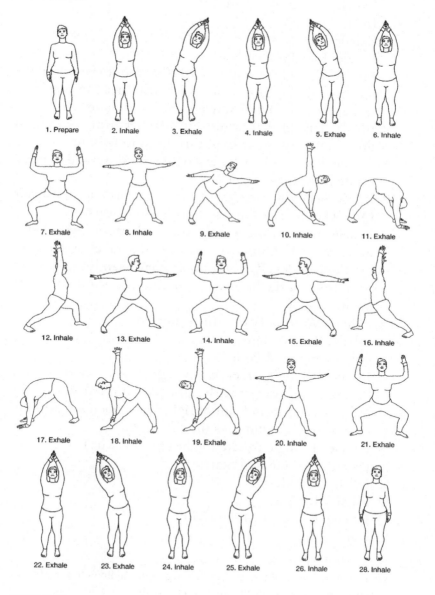

1. Prepare   2. Inhale   3. Exhale   4. Inhale   5. Exhale   6. Inhale

7. Exhale   8. Inhale   9. Exhale   10. Inhale   11. Exhale

12. Inhale   13. Exhale   14. Inhale   15. Exhale   16. Inhale

17. Exhale   18. Inhale   19. Exhale   20. Inhale   21. Exhale

22. Exhale   23. Exhale   24. Inhale   25. Exhale   26. Inhale   28. Inhale

56. Photo model Reed Kolber.

1. Begin in Mountain with hands by sides.
2. Inhale, sweep arms out to sides and overhead to Temple (interlace fingers, extend first fingers and thumbs).
3. Exhale, Crescent Moon left.[57]
4. Inhale, Temple.
5. Exhale, Crescent Moon right.
6. Inhale, Temple.
7. Exhale, Goddess.
8. Inhale, Five-Pointed Star.
9. Exhale, Triangle preparation left (left foot turns out, right foot slightly in, torso reaches left with head in line with spine, arms reach left staying parallel to floor).
10. Inhale, Triangle left (arms shift with left arm pointing to floor, right arm to ceiling, turn head to look up).
11. Exhale, Pyramid Pose (sweep right arm by ear and to floor, rotate hips to face left).
12. Inhale, bend the front knee and lift the torso up to Warrior One. Hands may come to hips or up by ears.
13. Exhale, open the torso to the side for Warrior Two. Hands may stay on hips or float to the sides, parallel to the floor.
14. Inhale, Goddess Pose. Option to have hands to the sides or in front of the heart in Namaste. Take three complete breaths.
15. Exhale, Warrior Two to the other side.
16. Inhale, Warrior One.
17. Exhale, Pyramid Pose.
18. Inhale, Triangle preparation right (eyes stay down for balance, prepare feet with right foot out, left in slightly, bring both arms in front of right knee, open left arm up, open shoulders and hips into Triangle).
19. Exhale, Triangle (rotate the head to look up).
20. Inhale, Five-Pointed Star.
21. Exhale, Goddess.
22. Inhale, Temple.
23. Exhale, Crescent Moon right.
24. Inhale, Temple.

---

57. Again, as described in Chapter 8, we are beginning all flows to the left side. To follow the pictures imagine that you are embodying the model. If you would prefer to begin to the right, simply reverse the written instructions.

25. Exhale, Crescent Moon left.
26. Inhale, Temple.
27. Sweep arms to sides slowly through the shape of the Full Moon, taking several breaths if desired.
28. Rest with one hand on belly, one hand on heart.
29. Repeat to the other side.

11

BREATH, PACING, AND MORE

I love to use the Moon Salutation as a way to launch a more extended flow. It's a great container for other poses.

~ Susan Kirinich, Kripalu Yoga Teacher

BREATH AND PACING

There is no one right way to breathe in this flow, and you may enjoy experimenting with different breath pacing. When practiced with one inhalation or exhalation per pose as described in the previous chapters, the flowing aspects of the Moon Salutation are emphasized. When the flow is done more slowly, taking several breaths per pose, you will more fully assimilate the inner experience of each pose.

It can be invigorating to breathe one breath per movement. As Kripalu Yoga Teacher Mary Lou Buck explains:

I absolutely love the breathing in the Moon Salutation. When I was learning it so that I could teach it to my students I got so invigorated from breathing deeply into the poses. It really opened my lungs. My students like to do it slowly. If I do it quickly they ask me to slow down.

Mary Lou also says that another option she uses is giving each posture a full in-and-out cycle of breath. She explains, "In this case my intention is to breathe in as I change positions and breathe out as I go into the posture. The inhalation is on the transition and the exhalation is the grounding." This deepens the holding of the pose.

For another variation, try experimenting with breathing out while changing positions, and then breathing in while holding, lengthening into the pose on the inhalation. Other practitioners like to flow in and out of the transitions between the poses multiple times before holding each pose for several breaths.

MORE WAYS TO VARY THE SEQUENCE

Many Yoga practitioners find their own ways to vary the Moon Salutation periodically to keep their practice interesting. Doing so reminds us that Yoga is not static, but alive, and may also provide ongoing challenge and interest to more physically advanced practitioners.

A wonderful way to vary the Moon Salutation is to insert additional poses into the flow. Be sure to do the same poses on each side for a balanced effect.[58]

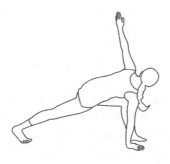

For example, from Lunge Pose extend the arm up and twist into Revolved Lunge Pose. Return back to Lunge Pose and continue the flow.

---

58. Photo model this chapter Laura Hernandez.

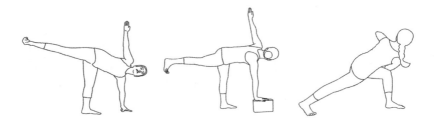

Another options is from Lunge Pose, come into Balancing Half Moon Pose. Next turn to Revolved Balancing Half Moon Pose. Then come into Twisting Crescent Lunge. Return the hands to the floor and come back into Lunge Pose.

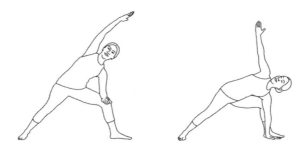

A great addition to the variations with high lunge is from Warrior Two, flow into Extended Side Angle. If flexibility allows, move into Extended Side Angle with Hand to Floor, then return to Warrior Two Pose. Continue with the flow as desired. Again, be sure to repeat any variations to both sides, either alternating sides, or in a circular flow.

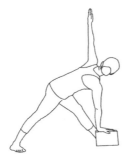
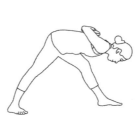

Another option is to insert Revolved Triangle after Triangle Pose... or place arms in Reverse Prayer Position when in Pyramid Pose.

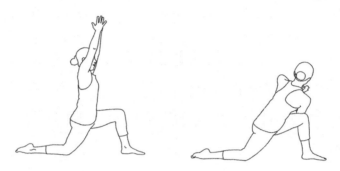

One might also insert Knee-Down Crescent Lunge or Twisting Crescent Lunge after Lunge Pose.

Infinite possibilities exist for incorporating poses into the Moon Salutation. The flow may also be done with hand *mudras* (or gestures), at a wall, in a chair, in a swimming pool, or on the floor. Please visit www.MoonSalutations.com for further inspiration.

PART THREE: FOUNDATIONS OF THE PRACTICE

12

CENTERING AND GROUNDING OURSELVES

The Moon Salutation meditation and practice have become a way of centering myself in my body and spirit. I affirm my beauty, power, love, and connection to all life in the universe. Incorporating the Yoga exercise into my day has also been a way of affirming my gratitude for a healthy body and my pledge to keep it strong and supple, ready for all that life has to offer.

~ Carol P. Christ, author, *Rebirth of the Goddess: Finding Meaning in Feminine Spirituality*

The Moon Salutation is fluid and gentle, grounded. It's like opening a flower. Women have the strength of childbearing, and I feel that in the Moon Salutation. It feels elegant, like the fullness of the moon.

~ Chris Keyser, student at the Berkeley YMCA

Practicing a series of poses with a clear beginning and clear end can create a profound ritual, a sense of having passed through sacred space. Moving slowly and steadily with the breath focuses the mind and centers our entire being in this moment and in the movement of the body. Over and over again when speaking with colleagues, students, and teachers, I would hear that practicing the Moon Salutation, any variation, grounds, centers, and empowers its practitioners.

As Patricia "Niti" Seip Martin, one of the Moon Salutation co-creators says, "The Moon Salutation is grounding simply because there is so much squatting. You put a lot of energy into the pelvis, the legs and feet." On a very basic level it awakens and strengthens the lower chakras. It opens the thighs wide and stretches the pelvis, the seat of power. Deepening into the body in the squats helps us to acknowledge and honor our physical embodiment.

Becoming more centered and grounded is something many of us in this busy world appreciate. Here's a story taken from my journal of how I released unnecessary worries in the process of demonstrating this flow:

Fall 1997: I'm teaching my first Moon Yoga for Women series at the Berkeley YMCA. After some warm-ups, I ask the students to squat or sit comfortably, telling them that I will now demonstrate the full Moon Salutation. "Don't worry about remembering the poses or their order," I say. "We'll have time for that later. Just watch for the essence of the flow." And I begin.

Many thoughts rush through my mind, but the steadiness and the strength of the flow quiet the thoughts. I hear my breath in the back of my throat, slow and steady. This grounds me. I see my body in the mirror moving into Crescent Moon, and I am reminded of other times I have seen that body in the mirror.

To me I am seeing the Goddess, embodying Her for my students. I drop into the impersonality and the dignity of that. I perform the poses as neutrally and yet completely as possible. I enjoy them fully.

When I finish I take a few extra breaths to bring my arms down full circle around my body, drawing the halo, the moon. I take a few breaths to feel the flow, and then I bring my hands in front of my heart in Namaste, open my eyes, and smile at the students. A blessing, a moment of connection.

Stepping to the side, I ask, "What did it feel like to watch this flow? What qualities did it embody to you?" I hear balanced, grounded, soothing. Someone comments that it looks more inward focused than the Sun Salutation, and asks if it feels that way to me. "Yes, it does," I respond.

Another participant notes that my voice has dropped. Before this demonstration my voice was higher. I know that she is right. Before the demonstration I had been worrying about how the class was going and whether I was making the right decisions along the way. Those worries are now gone, dissolved in the flow.

As women, we so often hold postures of submission, of fear, of stepping back from full participation. The Moon Salutation encourages us to release these constrictions and to invite every cell of our being to live full, something that is ultimately very empowering for our being. Sudha Carolyn Lundeen, RN and Yoga teacher trainer, points to the invitation we are given to expand into our fullest sense of self. "After sinking into the Goddess posture and feeling so open and grounded, it is fabulous to lengthen up and out into the 5-Pointed Star and get big ... be big ... be all that I can be. This is a radical stance for many women."

A strong heart energy ~ experienced often as radiant love ~ is felt in many of the poses of the Moon Salutation. These include Star, Triangle, Crescent Moon, and Temple Poses, as well as the final lowering of the arms through the shape of the full moon. As Yoga retreat leader Tracie Sage puts it, "When I do the Moon Salutation I feel very open-hearted, empowered, and creative, as though there's a lot of possibility in the world. I feel so much love."

The Moon Salutation can be especially empowering for those facing chronic or life-threatening illness. The ability to center in your own truth, coupled with the experience of an open heart, is a powerful combination to foster healing. Kripalu Yoga teacher Barbara Badger describes how she uses the Moon Salutation in classes for women with cancer:

I teach a Yoga class at the Wellness Community, a center that offers psychological support for cancer patients. The class is so unbelievably beautiful to me that I sometimes leave with tears flowing from every pore of my body. More than any other class, this is where I most become a vessel for the divine.

Women recovering from cancer close off to protect their energy field. This manifests physically in an inward posture where the elbows and shoulders roll forward and the chest rounds. The Moon Salutation asks you to stand and open. I have always found it healthy, empowering, and stabilizing.

I don't use the whole sequence with these women because many of them can't do the full series. Instead, I use different pieces to help them feel empowered. For women with lymphedema, I invite them to breathe deeply. The Goddess Pose is wonderful for women with cancer because it opens the groin, where so much of the immune and lymphatic system is located. Goddess Pose adds the openness in the groin to the openness in the arms so you are stimulating both areas.

We talk about how to take Yoga off of the mat and into your life. For example, after we do some moves from the Moon Salutation I might have them sit in their chairs, and then I ask them, "If you were in a doctor's office, what would be your first reaction? Of course it is to close in." So I tell them, "Remember what it's like to be here. Remember this empowerment." They tell me this is where they get their greatest benefit.

Illness is a turning point for many women, a gateway to new possibilities and new choices. Learning Moon Salutations at this time ~ whatever version or fragment thereof ~ supports women in going deeper, in choosing empowerment over collapse, courage over fear. It connects us to the field of energy in the heart and provides a way to feel both the vulnerability and power of love.

For many women, regardless of the diagnosis, reconnecting to our innate capacity for love is profoundly healing, whether the body is cured or not. No matter how brief your practice, no matter how short the flow you choose, always begin and end by coming home to yourself, by centering yourself in body, mind, spirit.

13

CELEBRATING ON THE FULL MOON

In the spring twilight
The full moon is shining:
Girls take their places
As though around an altar

And their feet move
Rhythmically, as tender
Feet of Cretan girls
Danced once around an

Altar of love, crushing a circle in the soft
Smooth flowing grass

~ Sappho

When I speak with others about the Moon Salutation, I hear over and over again that they love to practice and teach it on the full moon. Engaging in this flow at this time feels extra celebratory, extra joyful. We feel the moon's energy of fullness, knowing that others around the world are also celebrating on this night.

The word for full moon in Sanskrit is *purnima*. This word comes from the root "*purna*," meaning "wholesome, complete, or full." [59] The moon unites all humanity in the possibility of

---

59. So many possible definitions for the root word "purna" exist! Monier-Williams Sanskrit dictionary gives 30 separate possible translations for

grace and abundance. All people around the world, no matter where they live on the globe, see the moon as full on the same night. It is said in India that all month long we send our prayers and blessings to the moon and that on the full moon she sends them back.

Often I will ask women to share a favorite memory of the full moon, something that surprised or awed them. Common themes arise: The moon reflected over water, any water. The moon through the trees. Others say the Harvest Moon, so round and orange. One woman told me that she continued to be surprised by the moon as she moved to different locations around the world: "When I lived in Hawaii I thought there would never be anything as beautiful as the moon over a palm tree. Then I moved to the desert and I thought there would never be anything as beautiful as the moon rising over the mountain. Then I moved to California and I saw the moon in the redwoods."

A full-moon night is an excellent time to pause and reflect on the meaning and blessings of our lives. Often we notice gifts where we had previously seen only difficulties. The heart softens toward love, toward soulfulness, when seeing the full moon. This makes these nights especially potent for reflection, prayer, meditation, dance, and ecstasy.

Yoga educator Libby Cox shared this story of how dancing under the full moon enabled her to see her life in an entirely new way:

One of the most powerful experiences in my life was dancing in the light of the full moon on the beach in Bahia, Brazil. I was completely alone, the only human form on that beach. The moon was huge. Exhilarating. The light of the setting sun reflected nearby in tidal waters, right where the ocean meets the river.

---

this word as an adjective. The top 10 are: filled, complete, full, thorough, capable, strong, ended, abundant, satisfied, uttering this cry. To simplify the overwhelming number of definitions, I reached out to my "Sisters" group, a circle of women born in India, all Heartfulness meditators, and all of whom have much more familiarity with languages from the Indian sub-continent than I. And they responded that *purna* means "wholesome," "complete." I'll take their word for it.

As I danced, so much came together about the year I had just been through. Historically, I have always been a tomboy rather than a wild woman. That is, until the birth of my children. Before that there had been nothing succulent or resembling the dark goddesses in any way (except my love of the band Manic Panic and an unruly high-school boyfriend or two).

Yet this night with the moon showed me the true lunacy of this time in my life. I had birthed two babies, twins. I was as round and full as the Moon in the months before they were born. I howled like a ruddy Bhairavi during their birth. I bled. And bled. And met Kali.

I often sit now in self-conscious bitter sweetness in my 900-square-foot, certainly suitable apartment. I'm homebound more than I've ever been, oscillating between my attempts at busting hearts and minds in the few Yoga courses I still teach, and then coming home to watch teeth grow, hair grow. It's fantastic. And paradoxical.

At home I cultivate the best kind of heart-felt boredom I've ever known. Work is enchanting and soul feeding. I've spent most of my life wanting adventure and travel. Being at home is a new, slow-cooked pace.

I just watched a little clip of moonlight on the Brazilian ocean in a movie and started to cry. Then I looked over at the full, sweet faces on my boys and smiled. Here. My full-moon reflections. Them. The reflection and refraction of the light we've created. Okay.

Seeing the moon reminds us of the "okay-ness" of our lives. The moon speaks to us wordlessly. It speaks in presence, in awareness. But the message is always the same. "Okay. Your life is enough. It is perfect exactly as it is. Accept the gift of this life. Be open to receive."

When I can see life as a gift, no matter what, I have come into awareness of the meaning of the ancient *Purna Mantra* from the *Isha* and *Brihadaranyaka Upanishads*. I love this mantra for the way it so succinctly describes the fullness of our lives, the true meaning of full moon to me.

Here is the mantra, along with its translation:

Om purnamadah purnamidam
Purnaat purnamudachyate
Purnasya purnamaadaaya
Purnamevaavashishyate.

Om. That is perfect (full, whole). This is perfect.
From the perfect springs the perfect.
If the perfect is taken from the perfect,
The perfect always remains.

When our lives are full, more fullness arises. One may have a full life with partner and children, and a new baby is born, adding to the fullness. But what appears to be a "not-full" life is also part of the perfection. Being single. Losing a parent. Not being able to have a child. This life is perfect. This life is full.

The full moon informs our reflections as we sit in her presence, either on full-moon night itself, or when inviting her into our consciousness at other times. Inviting a painful or challenging situation into soft lunar awareness takes time and patience. Be gentle with yourself as you approach the questions of your life.

Yoga Instructor Beth Wadden has led a full-moon Yoga class every month since 1995, or 288 full-moon classes as of the time this book was completed. Here is her story:

I like to include special readings whenever I lead the Moon Salutation. I have a book on Arapaho full-moon stories for children, and another from Mexico. I abbreviate the stories and tell them at the beginning of class.

I attended a Yoga conference in 1996 that had the theme of the earth. We were all sliding around as if emerging from the sea ~ even in the convocations! That was a turning point for me. I realized that Yoga doesn't happen in carpeted studios with the proper lighting and a stereo. It's the awareness that we and the dolphins are related. I feel as if Native American Indians and also Indians in India viewed in that way. It didn't take place in the twice-vacuumed room but in the earth, in the mud, under the rain. So very often when you're doing the poses you begin to feel very celestial.

Whether you're practicing the Moon Salutation or the Sun Salutation, Five-Pointed Star or even side stretches; it's all very celestial. We let all of the elements breathe through the body. I just see it now as let the walls fade away, let the sky open and let's celebrate. We have a lovely time - and we howl at the moon!

Many Indian holidays fall on full moon. Here are just a few to guide your reflection. (Note that the dates vary each year according to the lunar cycle; check your calendar for exact dates.)

Pongal: Nurturing Water Full Moon. Comes in early winter. This is the day to honor the cleansing and life-giving power of water. Take a bath on this day, visit a sacred spring, or bring a bowl and sprinkle water on your sisters at a women's circle.

Holi: Full Moon of Color. Takes place in late winter. This is the Indian celebration of color, play, and dancing. On this day Indian people take to the streets to throw powdered paints and colors at each other, play with abandon, forgive each other for past grievances, and give gifts.

Buddha Jayanti: The Buddha is said to have been born, attained enlightenment, and died all on the full moon of late spring. Buddhists all over the world celebrate this day in honor of the joy of what the Buddha represents - the potential to rest in our fullness as truly awake beings.

Vat Purnima: Full Moon of the Banyan Tree. This is the day when women tie a string around a banyan tree with prayers of protection for their husbands.

Guru Purnima: Full Moon of the Teacher, which takes place in mid-summer. Here we honor the fullness of what we have received from our spiritual ancestors and guides; most importantly, the inner guide in the heart.

Rakhi Purnima: Full Moon of Brotherly Love, taking place in late summer. This is the day when sisters tie bracelets of protection on their brothers, celebrating the bond between women and our male friends everywhere.

These are just a few examples, and many other traditions also have lunar calendars, with special festivals to celebrate the special energies of the full, new or other days of the moon.

14

INVOKING EMPTINESS ON THE NEW MOON

Living a spiritual life means being willing to sit in the dark,
being willing not to know, to be terrified, to keep on sitting
and letting go.

~ China Galland, *The Longing for Darkness:*
Tara and the Black Madonna

There is humility in the emptiness of the new moon. The new moon is an experience of death, a vortex we enter and then return from each month. The moon cycles from full to new and back again, reminding us that everything that is good or bad in our lives must end, and that everything will be reborn. The cycles of the moon remind us of the cycles of nature, the heat and growth of summer giving way to the dark and quiet of winter.

Because the new moon appears so close to the sun in the sky, it becomes effectively invisible to the naked eye for three nights, the night before, during, and after the new moon. If you have never observed the moon when it was dark, it can be quite instructive to try. Look in the middle of the day, look at sunrise and sunset, look in the middle of the night ~ you won't see it. I remember when I did this almost 20 years ago. I realized that despite a beautiful clear, cloudless sky, despite being out in nature without any light pollution to obstruct the view, there really wasn't any moon. She really wasn't visible. This was amazing to me.

As much as our logical mind knows that the moon will return, another part of us wonders. What if she doesn't? What then? The mystical awe at this time of darkness is what inspired the ancient Jewish and Canaanite people to set up "watch people," criers who would literally stand on the edge of the city looking for the new moon and calling out when she appeared. This is the origin of the word calendar, from the Latin verb "*calare*," meaning to call out the new moon's appearance.

With electrical lights surrounding us and the 24/7 nature of our contemporary lives, it is almost impossible to imagine the impact that lunar phases would have had on pre-Edison peoples, but they were enormous. The first demarcation of time was based on the moon. Holidays were held on full and new moons, later adding in quarter moons as well, making four days of celebration per lunar month. This formed the basis of what came to be the week and the requisite rest on the Sabbath (previously quarter moons) when the calendar was separated from lunar rhythms and standardized with the sun instead.

Even more auspicious, and something we have perhaps lost even more completely, is the synchronization of women's menstrual cycles with the dark and light phases of the moon. The timing of the menstrual cycle is based on a woman's own internal clock, but also influenced by other factors, most importantly nighttime light, proximity to other women, stress, or being under-weight.

In an amazing synchronicity, the moon's light and dark phases match the cycle of human ovulation and menstruation, twenty-nine-and-a-half days. No other mammal has a menstrual cycle that so closely matches that of the moon.

Christiane Northrup, author of *Women's Bodies, Women's Wisdom*, cites research showing that when women are removed from artificial lighting and sleep instead under nocturnal light that mimics the moon's brightness, waxing, and waning, their cycles will shift so that they ovulate on the full moon and menstruate on the new moon. [60]

Biologically this makes sense. Women tend to need more rest when menstruating, and the dark of a moonless night lends itself

60. Christiane Northrup, *Women's Bodies, Women's Wisdom: Creating Physical and Emotional Health and Healing* (New York: Bantam Books, 1998), 104.

to early bedtime and deep sleep. Under the full moon, sleep is more difficult. We are naturally drawn to be awake, to meditate, to dance under the moon's light with friends and community. Timing ovulation with the full moon enhances fertility, as this is when a woman is most open to sex, and most likely to be able to become pregnant.

Just as menstruation has come to be seen as an unwelcome curse, so too the time of rest and quiet that is invited by the new moon has become uncomfortable in our contemporary society. To my mind, artificial light is something we would do well to minimize so as to allow a natural balance of sleep and other hormones to return. Minimizing artificial light also helps us attune to and enjoy the moon's natural phases, allowing them to remind us of our own cyclic need for rest. In an ideal world, new moon is a time of pause, a time to exhale and reflect. For many women it is an opportunity for renewal, emptying oneself out and preparing for rebirth.

Ayurveda Lifestyle Consultant Mirella Nicholson shared this story of how she created a new-moon ritual for healing of her inner feminine. Note that Mirella practices the Moon Salutation from the lineage of Vasant Lad, a slightly modified version of the Sun Salutation. And yet Mirella's intention to awaken the inner feminine and her openness to the energy of the moon create a similar experience of a lunar flow:

> Several years ago, I realized that I was completely out of touch with my lunar nature. I'm grateful for the solar energy that gave me the strength I needed to take care of my family, but I knew something was missing. I was struggling in an abusive marriage and completely shut off from my emotions.
>
> I decided to embark on an adventure. Beginning on a new moon, I flowed through eleven rounds of the Moon Salutation each night and then chanted the moon mantra "Om Som Somaya Namaha" 108 times. This new-moon sadhana continued every night until the following new moon. The practice had a beautiful soft, fluid, and receptive quality to it that provided a balance to the harshness of my daily life at the time. I had come to believe that being soft and receptive wasn't safe.

The moon began to reveal her lessons to me, and I gradually found my way back to myself. Each new moon I would plant my intentions. I wanted to be myself and to live wholeheartedly. I wanted a life of joy and ease. I lovingly tended those seeds of intention every evening as I practiced. At the full moon I would allow the light of the moon to illuminate for me all the patterns and beliefs that were blocking me from the life I wanted. I would ask for Divine Mother's help in releasing those things.

My whole world has changed since I began the practice. I eventually ended my abusive, dysfunctional marriage. My life has become like a garden. There is more fluidity where before there was rigidity. I continue to celebrate each new moon and I lead new-moon workshops to share what I learned.

15

POEM ~ MEDITATION ON THE MOON SALUTATION

I remember vividly the time I first felt the vibrant energy of the earth. I was a teenager and had hiked through the fields up a hill behind my house to a soft, cool patch between two ponds. I lay down and felt the earth pressing against me, wordlessly sending her presence into my heart. From her vast reserves she filled me with steadiness, courage, and peace. This was the same hill I dreamed of in my twenties as shared at the beginning of this book, the hill that I saw in my dream as glowing with light.

Since the time of my teens I have found many ways of tapping into this awe-inspiring source. One is through contemplating the full moon. Another is through the practice of Moon Salutations. Early in my journey with the Moon Salutation I was inspired to write a meditation that described my inner experience of the poses and of the sequence overall. Many practitioners have found that this meditation deepens their experience of the flow.[61]

I offer this poem as a gift for your practice. I invite you to read it and receive its message for you. Even more, I invite you to experience the full circular Moon Salutation (with high or low lunges) while listening to the words. You can download an audio recording from www.MoonSalutations.com.

---

61. An earlier version of this poem appears in Carol P. Christ, *She Who Changes: Re-Imagining the Divine in the World* (New York: Palgrave Macmillan, 2003), 241-242. A different version appeared in my book *The Moon Salutation: Expression of the Feminine in Body, Psyche, Spirit* (Emeryville, CA: Yogeshwari Arts, 2000), 89-90.

MEDITATION ON THE MOON SALUTATION

*I stand tall, heart open to the world, body full and present in
all of its beauty.*
I open my arms wide to bring all of life into my being.
*My arms form a temple above me, protecting and shelter-
ing me.*
I know that I am on holy ground.

*Yielding now, softening, my body takes the shape of the cres-
cent moon.*
*Rising up and bending to the other side, I know that my soft-
ness is my strength.*
I am tested, but not broken.

I step wide now into a squat.
*Mother Earth's ferocious powers rise up through my strong legs,
hips, and back.*
*As mother, I give birth to all that is, caring for and protecting
all life.*

*Straightening arms and legs I am a star ~ I am the
universe.*
Planets and galaxies whirl within me.
I radiate light in all directions.

Supple and yielding again, I stretch to the side,
Allowing my body to be a vehicle for change in this world.
I rotate my arms and look up.
I reach, yearning and striving, yet rest, accepting fully.

Turning to Pyramid Pose I become quiet.
*Head to knee, I submit to the inner workings of my own
being.*

I stretch long and feel again the glorious length of my body.
I ask for blessings and protection on my path.

*Turning now, I touch the earth, hands on the blessed mother,
strong and steady. Gratefully and tenderly, I bow my head.*

Coming into a squat, I am connected with all animal and
   plant life.
My yoni is open and close to the earth,
I am the dark moon.
For three days and nights I will stay here.
I know my body's ability give birth, to love, to work, to pray.
I resolve to hold all of these activities as sacred.

Reemerging now I retrace my steps.
Dear Earth, You have been with me when I needed comfort,
Given me wisdom when I was in pain.
I pray I may do the same for you.

Turning to the side, I see the moon shining on my path,
I am here, divine spirit, to do your bidding.

I am restored and nourished.
I feel my breath, my bones, my flesh.

I know the world with all its sorrow and pain and I am not
   afraid.
I know myself with all of my sorrow and pain and I am not
   afraid.

I open to love and compassion.
I embrace my ferocity, my sexuality, my power.

As I move and bend, my heart stays open to the world.
I feel the sweet stillness, always present within me.

I am the full moon.
I am whole.
I am complete.
I am light and dark.
I am the inside and the outside.
I am one with all.

Om Shanti

PART FOUR: NURTURING A WOMAN'S BODY

16

COOLING, OPENING, AND NOURISHING

The female orientation is to start with nourishing rather than challenging. It's a juicy, sensuous, feeling orientation.

~ Tanya Davis, Former Kripalu Programs Director

Feminine embodiment requires nourishment, nurturing. As women go through hormonal and physical changes, our bodies as well as our Yoga practice must adapt to these changes. While a man's physiology is more constant, a woman's body changes with monthly hormonal shifts as well as the more dramatic changes of childbearing and menopause. While a woman's body may need rest during menstruation, menopause, and early pregnancy, the changes in and of themselves create a need to pause, nourish the body, and integrate the transition.

Even beyond this inherent need for nourishment, women today face an epidemic of overwork, exhaustion, and resulting mood disorders. Women are primed to over-give in careers and relationships. Mothers face the relentless demands of childrearing in a culture that does not fully support parents and children, and even in dual-parent households, women carry a disproportionate burden of the childcare. Sadly, many of us never saw good models of healthy rest during menstruation, early pregnancy, menopause, or simply as needed to bring happiness.

Chronic fatigue, insomnia, anxiety, and depression all result from over-giving. Caring for others can be nurturing and health promoting, but when it's all you have time for, illness results. Taking care of ourselves is essential for every other health improvement. Relaxation is the first ingredient of self-care and Yoga is one of the best ways to address the exhaustion that accompanies so many women's lives.

COOLING THE BODY

In many ways, menstruation, menopause, and early pregnancy are similar energetically. During these times, women need a Yoga practice that is cooling and tranquilizing for the nervous system. In both Ayurvedic and Chinese medicine, menstruation and menopause are considered to generate excess heat in the body. In menstruation, this is due to hormonal changes and to the work needed to release the menstrual tissue from the body. In menopause, this is due to hormonal fluctuations and adjustments. Fluctuating hormones can also create excess heat during pregnancy. When there is excess heat, the body will feel more tired and need more rest.

It's not always necessary for a woman to have a gentle practice. On days when she has high energy, it is important for her to practice more vigorously and exercise aerobically to benefit her general health. These times include the middle of the menstrual cycle, adolescence, high-energy days during menopause, and the post-menopausal years.[62] At these times both the Moon and Sun Salutations will be beneficial.

The yogic way of understanding whether a pose is cooling and calming or heating and stimulating is contained in the Ayurvedic principle of *brhmana* and *langhana*. All poses are seen as existing along a spectrum from very brhmana, or heating, to very langhana, or cooling.[63] This concept is critical to understanding the energetic effect of the Sun and Moon Salutations. The heating or cooling nature of a pose depends on multiple factors, including the amount of muscular exertion required, whether the pose

---

62. Linda Sparrowe and Patricia Walden, *The Woman's Book of Yoga and Health: A Lifelong Guide to Wellness* (Boston, MA: Shambhala, 2002).

63. Richard Miller, "The Psychophysiology of Respiration: Eastern and Western Perspectives," *The Journal of the International Association of Yoga Therapists* 2, no. 1 (1991).

naturally emphasizes inhalation or exhalation, and other subtle influences on the nervous system.

Heating poses include backbends, arm balances, and most standing poses. Richard Miller, Founder of iRest Yoga Nidra, explains: "These poses activate the sympathetic nervous system, the mechanisms of excitation in the body." [64] Backbends are heating because they "encourage a full and lengthy inhalation, making it slightly more difficult to exhale." [65] Cooling poses include forward bends, side bends, and twists. Due to the action on the spine, these postures naturally encourage a lengthy and deep exhalation. There is a deep stillness at the end of the exhalation. This emphasis on exhalation is tranquilizing for the body. It activates the parasympathetic nervous system, the responses of relaxation, rest, and ease.[66]

In carefully looking at the Sun Salutation, we see that its overall effect is brhmana, or heating.[67] While it contains both forward and backward bends, more of the poses are backward bends. In addition, Downward Facing Dog, technically a forward bend, is actually heating for the body due to the fact that it is a partial arm balance.

Moon Salutations, in contrast, contain primarily side bends and forward bends. The only backbend, Lunge Pose (or Warrior One in the high lunge version), is a very gentle backbend. While the Goddess Pose requires strength in the thighs and is thus heating, it is outnumbered by the other more cooling poses. Thus, the overall effect of the Moon Salutation is langhana, or cooling. For these reasons, the Sun Salutation is more beneficial for times when the nervous system is in need of energizing, while Moon Salutations are more beneficial for times when the nervous system is in need of soothing and grounding.

---

64. Ibid.
65. Ibid.
66. Ibid.
67. Miller, personal communication, July 2, 1999.

OPENING THE HIPS AND PELVIS

At nearly all times in a woman's life cycle, it is beneficial to open the hips and pelvis. Hip-opening poses massage the ovaries and uterus while relaxing the entire pelvic area. [68] This maintains mobility of the organs, supports healthy hormonal function and fertility, and strengthens the abdominal wall and pelvic floor. Deep breathing while in these poses extends the benefits of stretching and massage to the organs. It can prevent adhesions between the pelvic organs and the abdominal wall by increasing circulation and encouraging the natural gliding action between adjacent tissues. Deep breathing also relaxes the body to reduce stress.

Moon Salutations are full of hip openers, as its creators intentionally used these poses to massage and open the female body. Crescent Moon and Triangle are side-bending poses that also stretch across the front of the belly and into the internal organs. Goddess Pose opens the inner thighs widely and encourages the yoni (the birth canal and entire genital region) to relax. For those dropping into the low lunging poses, Side Lunge opens the muscles across the inner thigh and groin, while Full Squat is a hip opener that deeply relaxes the hips and pelvic floor.

While these poses are beneficial for a woman at all times in her life cycle, they are particularly useful during menstruation, pregnancy, and menopause. During menstruation, heaviness in the belly and thighs is relieved by hip-opening poses. During pregnancy, hip openers help relax the pelvic floor, preparing the mother to relax and open deeply during labor.[69] After menopause, maintaining a healthy blood flow to the pelvis can be an important factor in keeping vaginal tissues vital and juicy. Deep breathing into the pelvis and maintaining healthy pelvic muscles helps prevent pelvic prolapse.

One exception to the hip-opening rule is postpartum, when it is important to rebuild the pelvic floor and abdominal tone in general. More beneficial movements during this period are

---

68. Geeta Iyengar, *Yoga: A Gem for Women* (2013, reprint, New Delhi, India: Allied Publishers Pvt. Limited).
69. Ibid.

properly-performed kegel exercises and specific abdominal strengtheners.[70]

RESTORATIVE POSES FOR MOON TIME

Moon Time is any time you are in need of a little more nurturing, a little more rest. Restorative poses soothe tired nerves as well as relax the body during menstruation, menopause, or early pregnancy. The sequence of poses in this section is an adjunct to the Moon Salutation, a sequence that you can do when you are too tired for standing poses. You may find that starting your practice with a restorative sequence rejuvenates you so much that you are ready to practice standing poses immediately after. Or the restorative poses may be used as a stand-alone practice all on their own, especially on days when you are extremely tired.

Moving the body into these different positions is highly beneficial. The poses give the internal organs a beautiful massage and open the energy meridians. They stimulate the flow of blood and lymph. This prevents stagnation of the body, even as you rest deeply. Through practicing restorative poses we can learn to find pleasure in the simple act of rest.

This sequence was created by Stacey Louise, Child and Teen Yoga Therapist, who shares her thoughts about the nurturing value of restorative Yoga:

> *Restorative poses offer a nurturing, soft space for women to take time out and connect within. Adapting the poses to wide leg variations will allow more nurturing space for the belly. Using props (bolsters, bricks, straps, blankets, eye pillows, and soothing music) will allow the practitioner to feel that she is safe and supported. She can let go fully.*

---

70. Sparrowe and Walden, *The Woman's Book of Yoga and Health*. Also note that even without doing kegels, deep belly breathing can help to reverse diastasis recti (separated abdominal muscles after childbirth) and may also help prevent incontinence and organ prolapse.

1. Child's Pose

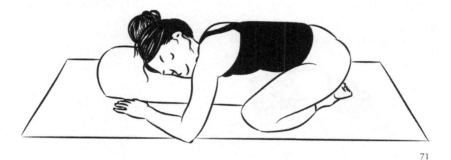

71

- Knees wide apart
- Bolster at mid thigh and under chest
- Turn head to one side and relax shoulder

Duration: 2-5 minutes
Benefit: Eases cramping and lower back pain; provides deep rest

2. Child Twist

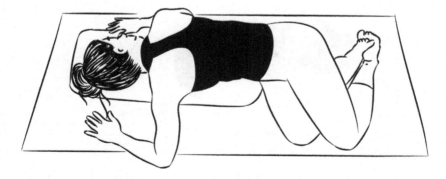

- A bolster under the chest
- Hands frame the bolster
- Knees to one side, head faces to the other side

---

71. Photo model restorative poses, Stacey Louise.

Duration: 2-5 minutes each side
Benefit: Gentle detoxifying twist without hurting the belly

3. Pigeon Pose

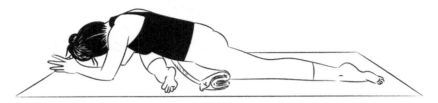

- A rolled blanket under the front hip and back thigh

- Optional: Rest the chest against a bolster or cushion (not pictured)

- Relax the shoulders

Duration: 2-5 minutes each side
Benefit: Eases cramping and decreases irritability

4. Supine Butterfly Pose

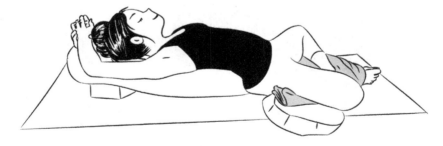

- A bolster with a block or blanket under it creating an incline. Adjust with additional blankets or blocks as needed to make the incline higher or lower. Some practitioners will be more supported with a blanket under the bolster where the shoulders are so that the spine is in alignment. There should be no discomfort in your back at any point.

- A blanket around the feet and cushions under the thighs. Do not let the thighs open too deeply.

- Hands on belly or resting over the head.

Duration: 5-10 minutes
Benefit: Opens the uterus to help with an easeful flow; feminine surrender; opens the hips wide; provides deep rest

5. Wide Legs Up The Wall

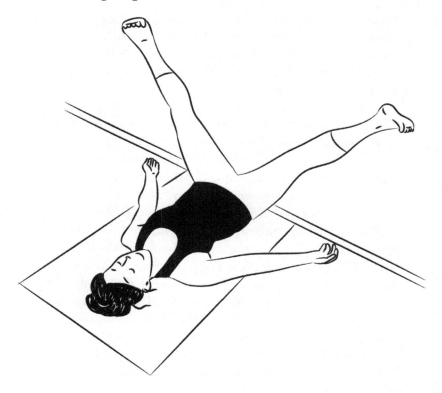

- Lie with the hips close to the wall

- Keep them floor level

- Open the legs into a wide V

- Hands on belly or by the side

Duration: 5-10 minutes

Benefit: Improves circulation; deep rest

▸   ▸   ▸

While opening the hips wide has physiological benefits, it also opens us to an entirely new mode of being. When the thighs and kneecaps face forward as in the Sun Salutation, we're ready to step ahead and take on life. But when the thighs turn out we open to a whole new realm of experience. We feel, we slow down, we explore. Activities done with open thighs include dancing, making love, and birthing babies.

Many practitioners I spoke with noted how dropping into the hips and opening sideways invited an entirely different psychological orientation. Yoga Therapist and author Jenny Berthiaume recounts how the Moon Salutation opens her to a spiraling, labyrinth-like experience:

> *The weekend before Halloween, I returned from a workshop where we moved our hips - a lot. We discussed the moon and cycles and all things deeply feminine. In the week that followed I led a luscious, delicious, move your pelvis like you mean it experience in all my classes.*
>
> *And we did the Moon Salutation. The flowing, strong and sacred Moon Salutation. As I taught it again and again over the course of the week, I could for the first time really FEEL how it is oh so different from the linear Sun Salutation we do again and again. Front foot back, right and left. Straight plank, straight arms. Again and again.*
>
> *The glorious FREEDOM of the Moon Salutation! The almost disorienting nature of spiraling around like the labyrinth that is labor and birth and parenting! I like to get lost in the movements, experiencing the meditative muscle memory of my body flowing in a circle.*

As the hips open physically, we experience a new realm of being psychologically. Once again the Moon Salutation beckons us beyond the physical body into an exploration of psyche and spirit.

17

HONORING MENSTRUATION

Many women feel naturally quieter and more reflective on their periods. This makes sense, as on a physical level, the menstrual period is a release, a physical letting go of the blood and nutrients that are not needed to support a baby. It takes work to expel blood and tissues from the uterus. No wonder women are a bit tired at this time.

Your periods are natural. They are a sign that your body is ready to have a baby. They are a good thing, an indication of health and vitality. And yet, energetically, menstruation is a time of death. The ovum is literally dying, and a woman thus becomes more attuned to those inherent processes of death and release that are part of life. This is a lot to integrate, whether or not you are wanting to become pregnant. Giving this process space leads to peacefulness and balance. Going against the flow through over-activity creates agitation, cramping, and other signs of discomfort.

There was wisdom in ancient traditions that encouraged rest, seclusion, and gathering with other women on one's period. Native American women gathered in the moon lodge, Hebrew women in the red tent, and Hindu women with sisters and friends in combined families and extended village networks.[72]

Being released from one's normal duties supports healthy menstruation. Collective households made it easier for women to have time off from housework when needed and provided

---

72. Of course these customs all varied greatly by tribe, geographic location, caste, level of education, historical period, etc.

companionship in quieter times. In many traditional cultures, menstrual blood was revered for its life-giving properties and menstrual seclusion was a time for women to rest, play, and gather their sacred energy.

Sadly, what may have been beneficial and balancing for women became over-limiting, constrictive, and degrading. Menstrual taboos put a heavy burden and negative stigma on women worldwide. In differing eras of almost every religion across the globe, superstition and lack of knowledge led to menstruating women being seen as unclean, harmful to men or unborn babies, and often much worse. Sadly, in many places those stigmas still exist.

The tissue leaving your body is not full of "toxins" as was previously thought. While it is no longer needed to grow a baby, menstrual flow is actually rich in nutrients (nitrogen, phosphorous, and potassium) and even stem cells, progenitor cells that have the potential to grow into other cell types needed by the body.[73] For this reason, many women swear that their menstrual blood is the best plant fertilizer available.

The natural time of quiet that comes with the shedding of blood and tissue corresponds also with a time of heightened dreams. Scientists measuring women's dreams over the menstrual cycle have found that "women's dreams are more frequent and often more vivid during the premenstrual and menstrual phases of their cycles."[74] Many women believe they are more spiritually attuned on their periods, and many traditional cultures support this view.

In our culture, a deep respect for the power of the body to give birth and its related monthly changes were replaced with shame. I personally hid my first period from my mom. I was so embarrassed by my body and its bleeding that I hid my bloody underwear in a drawer. Disconnected emotionally from my mother, it never occurred to me to tell her, or to ask her to buy me menstrual pads. Somehow she found the underwear in the

---

73. Lijun Chen, Jingjing Qu, and Charlie Xiang. "The Multi-functional Roles of Menstrual Blood-derived Stem Cells in Regenerative Medicine." *Stem Cell Research and Therapy* 10 (2019). https://www.ncbi.nlm.nih.gov/pmc/articles/PMC6318883/ (accessed May 13, 2019)

74. Christiane Northrup, *Women's Bodies, Women's Wisdom,* 105.

drawer and looked at me in surprise. "Why didn't you tell me?" she asked. I felt utterly ashamed.

Gradually I came to accept my periods, and to do what was needed to manage them. I learned Yoga poses that opened and stretched the belly and low back, noticeably relieving the cramps. I found that the Moon Salutation often felt good when I was bleeding, but at other times I just wanted to lie on the floor and stretch gently or do restorative poses. But it would be several decades longer before I learned to embrace menstruation. Despite everything I had learned and practiced, my cramps didn't really improve until I surrendered to rest.

The tipping point in my menstrual journey came in my mid-40s. I began to have severe sacroiliac pain that attacked when I got my period, subsided slightly about two weeks later, and returned again with a vengeance on the next cycle. Nine months later I had tried everything I could think of to relieve the pain and seen multiple health-care practitioners, but nothing was working.

I began to lie on the couch for all meals, draping my body over soft pillows, propping myself up on my left arm and eating with the right. I told my husband about the menstrual rituals of women being relieved of household duties on their periods. He was happy to help and did the bulk of the housework for the two or three heavy days of my flow. I felt like a queen and truly looked forward to these times. I saved up special movies to watch on my period and looked for other fun things to do with friends. I found that when I relaxed fully on one period, the cramps would be lighter the next. My back improved, and I continued to practice deep menstrual rest until I entered menopause a decade later.

Because the Moon Salutation is oriented toward the female body and life cycle, it helps to bring menstruation into the open, where any shame or awkwardness is released and participants experience mutual honoring instead. Yoga retreat leader Tracie Sage teaches the Moon Salutation in a special series on women's health. She first has participants arrange themselves in a circle according to their stage of life. Within the circle, those who are of menstruating age arrange themselves by day of cycle. Tracie then has the women introduce themselves and learn the Moon Salutation arranged this way in the circle:

Having shared like that, the women are very connected. I get chills even thinking about it. When we come into Goddess Pose there's a strong sense of unity. When we come into full Squat it feels as though we're connected to each other and to the cycles of a woman's life. Somehow, from that it feels as though we're connected to the universe. I think it is fabulous and I think the women get as big of a charge out of it as I do.

Enjoy your periods as a time of rest and a time to cherish yourself. You are a part of this earth and part of the cycles of nature. All of nature needs to take time to rest, and this is yours. Pamper yourself with extra meditation, writing in your journal, gentle Yoga stretches, and conversations with friends. If you have dreams, write them down. If it feels good to walk in nature, do that. If it feels good to take a Yoga class, do that.

Tune in to whatever your body needs. Listen and ask inwardly, and follow the guidance you receive. Once you know what will feel good to you, ask the people around you to support you. Invite them to do something special and nourishing for you, or to take on a little more of the housework while you rest. While not all women are tired during their periods, in general Yoga practice at this time should be gentler and softer than during the rest of the month. If you have cramps, practice belly down poses such as boat, bow, or cobra to give a shiatsu-like effect. If you have lower back pain, practice gentle forward bends, such as wide legged forward bend with your head draped on a pillow.

During menstruation, you may be too exhausted to practice any standing poses at all. A restorative sequence may be more appropriate. For deep rest, practice the poses shown in Chapter 16 then take a 30-minute nap. Often, a restorative sequence followed by a nap will completely refresh the body during menstruation.

For those who would like to do standing poses, the Moon Salutation offers an excellent sequence. Many of the poses in this flow are those considered most beneficial for menstruation, such as Triangle and Crescent Moon. Pyramid Pose and Full Squat release tension in the lower back, helping to relieve pain in this area. Go through the Moon Salutation very slowly, breathing into and enjoying each of the poses. Then turn to some gentle floor stretches to complete your practice, ending again with a nap, or at a minimum a 10-minute Relaxation Pose.

A Menarche Ritual for Teen Girls

Many women are experimenting with new menarche rituals for teen girls as a way to break the cycle of shame. These women have a goal of empowering the next generation for a healthier start than my generation had. Stacey Louise, Child and Teen Yoga Therapist, describes how she guides teen girls through the rites of passage into womanhood:

> *I could see that I had struggled for almost two decades through painful menstrual cycles because I had played victim to the taboo and dishonoring of menstruation in our modern culture.*
>
> *I decided to create a series for the girls to encourage a menarche (first menstruation) ritual, bringing it into my Yoga For Teen Girls class. I ask the girls in my series how they would like to be celebrated at menarche. Options include having a day off from school; being pampered with a foot rub, facial, or hair treatment; starting a journal; or receiving a piece of jewelry.*
>
> *I tell them stories from Eastern and Indigenous traditions that recognize menstruation as a time of heightened spirituality. I tell them that I have learned ~ in my own body and from my Yoga therapy clients ~ that resting on one's period lightens the cramps over time.*
>
> *I apologize on behalf of all of the women in their lives who failed to talk openly with them about menstruation. I let them know it is probably because they themselves didn't have an open introduction to their cycle. I let them know it's OK to feel awkward talking about menstruation, that it may seem weird, rude or gross, but that it's only because we have been conditioned to feel that way.*
>
> *I teach them restorative and other poses for menstruation. I encourage journaling and praise rest.*

18

SUPPORTING A HEALTHY PREGNANCY AND BIRTH

Whether you've birthed a child, a business, a work of art, or whether you're birthing your spiritual Self, it's all included. It's all part of our creative powers.

~ Deva Parnell, Former Senior Program Teacher, Kripalu Center

Pregnancy is a time of great spiritual and psychological opening. Pregnant women eat for two, sleep for two, and breathe for two, all while experiencing dramatic physical and emotional transformations. Yoga provides potent means to support optimal wellness during what can be an exciting but often physically grueling transition. Yoga invites a woman to connect to her growing body, her baby, and her path as a mother.

I didn't carry a child in this lifetime, but I watched many friends and my sister do so, and I saw repeatedly what a powerful transformative experience it is. I do believe I've had children in other lifetimes, and I relate closely to the experience of being a mother. I remember the tears of awe and joy my sister shed often in the first few weeks of caring for her newborn. I felt them too, in visiting her and helping care for my niece.

In the Divine Feminine Leadership Training I offered last year we spent an evening focusing on our relationship to our female bodies. I was struck that most of what was shared was difficult and painful ~ all the trauma and challenges that can come with feminine embodiment. And so I asked, "What are the positive aspects of having a female body?" Yoga Teacher and Massage Therapist Deah Jenkins immediately spoke, describing what a miracle it was to have had a child. She later shared with me the journal entry she wrote after our session that night:

> I am thankful for the miracle of my feminine body! The love and passion with my husband created a spark that ignited life to a beautiful soul who was ready to shine bright in this world. I am thankful for the miracle of her life force that grew inside of me. I am honored and empowered to consciously mother, protect, and teach.

The Moon Salutation was created to honor this generative, deeply creative process of birth. Arisika Razak, M.P.H., former Chair and Professor Emerita of Women's Spirituality and an inner city nurse midwife of 20 years, immediately noticed this when she was first taught the Moon Salutation:

> When I first saw the Moon Salutation, I felt that finally someone had created something that honored the female body. Here was something I could relate to. Some postures of the Sun Salutation are prohibited during pregnancy and menstruation. However the Moon Salutation has postures that can be done when you're menstruating or during some parts of pregnancy. And immediately I saw that the squatting posture is also a birthing posture. These poses are tied to women's innate physicality. The memory of that is held both within the body and within many "traditional" cultures of color ~ village cultures all over the world ~ where women still remember and still experience birth in the squatting position.

Arisika elaborated that for her, the Moon Salutation provided relief from the birth-denying, birth-denigrating aspects of some strands of Hinduism and Buddhism:

> I've been at conferences where Buddhist texts were shared that described the stench of being in the womb and the heat and the disgust experienced by the fetus. Some texts even say

that the Buddha wasn't in his mother's womb at all, but that he gestated in some sort of a crystal vase in his mother's body, and that he didn't even come out of that "nasty" vagina, but emerged from an opening in her side so as not to be polluted. Here we see virgin birth again, as if there were something wrong with coming through the vagina, or yoni.

So I was deeply moved to find a place where the female body was honored as a source, a site of sacredness. For me, the Moon Salutation is a woman-honoring, woman-reverencing process.

Arisika also notes that while not all women give birth, the majority still do. For many, this is a deeply spiritually transformative experience. She continues:

I know that in the developed world we do so many things as women. I'm not trying to essentialize and say that all women should have children or should want to have children. But most of the world's women still do have children today. And for many, many women, this is a deeply spiritual experience. It is deeply, deeply spiritual to carry a child, especially a wanted child. It is a deeply, deeply spiritual act to conceive and to form this union in the body.

At the moment when I was pushing, right before my son was born, I felt that I had a universe between my legs. This echoes the painting I've seen of Mother Kali giving birth to the universe. He is coming out hands above head in perfect prayer position. Right before my child was born there was a sense of all the possibilities, all the potential that could come into being with this child.

▼ ▼ ▼

During the first three months of pregnancy, many women are tired and need extra rest. In this early part of pregnancy, there is a high risk of miscarriage, and it is important that if you feel tired you not over-exert. Later the fetus becomes better established in the womb and you will feel stronger again. Pay attention to your energy level and adjust accordingly.

When you're ready for standing poses, the Moon Salutation is an excellent sequence. Again, many of its poses are those most often recommended for pregnancy. Hip openers are particularly beneficial at this time, and the Full Squat is often given as the most beneficial and important pose for pregnancy. Doing squats as in the Moon Salutation helps to restore or maintain the normal function of the body to open in the hips. Arisika Razak notes, "In cultures where squatting is still the normative way of sitting rather than sitting on a chair, birth is easier." Goddess Pose will help to strengthen the thighs and core of the body, preparing you for the marathon of labor and delivery. Crescent Moon and Triangle Poses open the ribs and torso, creating room for your baby to grow and for you to breathe.

Unlike the Sun Salutation, which contains several poses contraindicated during pregnancy (Standing Backbend, Standing Forward Bend, and Cobra), all the poses of the Moon Salutation are safe and beneficial for most pregnant women. Pyramid Pose is actually one of the few standing forward bends in which the belly is not constricted and which is thus accessible during pregnancy.

Practicing the Moon Salutation and Yoga in general during pregnancy can generate confidence and wellbeing. Cake designer and Heartfulness practitioner Chaitra Makam was in her ninth month of pregnancy, just 10 days from her due date, when she participated in a Yoga class that I taught at the Heartfulness Meditation Center we both attended. This was not a prenatal class but an all-levels class. Knowing how pregnant she was and wanting to support her upcoming labor, I prepared a special class in her honor. The session included a gentle variation of the Moon Salutation along with other standing, squatting, and sitting poses intended to create space in the pelvis and ribs while also being accessible and safe for Chaitra. Chaitra had recently fallen and had a badly swollen knee, thus we needed to avoid all poses on hands and knees, usually a common position in prenatal classes.

Here is what Chaitra had to say looking back two years later about her practice of Yoga during pregnancy and that class in particular:

Yoga helped me to feel calmer in my mind. When I was doing Yoga I could focus on the positive aspects of pregnancy rather than just the pains and irritations that come up from all of the hormones. Toward the end of pregnancy Yoga definitely helped in opening my pelvis, but even more it helped with lower back pain. Sleep became really difficult at the end of pregnancy. My stomach was so big I could hardly turn over. I saw a huge difference with Yoga, that when I practiced I was able to sleep continuously for several hours with no back pain.

That class right before my delivery definitely boosted my confidence. At that time certain poses were difficult, but I thought, "If I can do that, I can do anything." In my previous pregnancy I hadn't done Yoga, but I was more flexible the second time than in my previous pregnancy, because of the Yoga.

On that day the rest of the class also got the benefit of the prenatal, hip-opening session. Even more, the group's openness to a prenatal class explicitly designed for Chaitra was a way to celebrate and encourage her for the labor to come.

The Moon Salutation can also help pregnant women tune in to their intuition and protectiveness and to evoke their collective strength together. Yoga teacher Martha Chabinsky describes how she draws on the Moon Salutation in her prenatal classes:

I use the Moon Salutation in most of my classes as a warm-up, but I especially like it for my prenatal classes. In my mind there is nothing more beautiful than an 8-9 month pregnant woman in the Full Squat with her hands in Namaste.

As participants move through the posture flow, they naturally bond with each other and see that their seemingly unique experience is actually universal.

In particular, Goddess Pose helps them recognize their inherent strength and power. I call it the "Don't mess with me" pose, which makes them laugh. They already feel protective of their unborn babies, and by giving them an opportunity to join together and mirror one another, they stand taller, rooted in their truth.

When doing the squats we talk about tuning in to their intuition regarding birthing options. We use sound during that part of the salutation to experience how the earth supports them in this natural process of bringing life into the world.

Not all women are able to practice the Moon Salutation during pregnancy. Women with special needs or those who experience extreme pain or joint instability may do better with a different sequence or simply with rest. Adaptive Yoga Instructor Erin Dowd shared the following story of her experience:

At the end of my pregnancy, all I could do was Supta Baddha Konasana *(Supine Butterfly Pose, shown in Chapter 16). I would prop myself up on pillows, then rest in that pose, sleep in that pose, everything. I did not lie down for a couple of months. I couldn't even lie on my side. I thought to myself, "I can't wait for this birth to happen!" I was in so much pain I could hardly walk. I had women who would see me in the grocery store and help me out. They would say, "I remember the pain."*

Because I had a cesarean, I needed to recover. In time I was able to move through the whole Moon Salutation again. My favorite and most common place to practice would be at the diaper-changing table with my baby. While she was drying off between diapers I'd use the diaper table as a prop. I would keep an eye on her and she always had her eyes on me - her first exposure to Yoga.

Solidarity between women is probably nowhere more needed than in pregnancy, childbirth, and child-rearing. I send a prayer to all those who desire to parent and to all those who are currently parenting. I believe our world does not do enough to support parents and children, and also that parenting is the most critical work on the planet. Nothing is more important than raising conscious, loving children - nothing more needed than tender parenting. The Moon Salutation carries this fierce understanding of the value of motherhood, and of protecting our own and each other's children.

19

HEALING THE WOUNDS OF MISCARRIAGE, STILLBIRTH, AND INFERTILITY

It's impossible to approach birth without also approaching death. Birth and death, for better or worse, are closely linked gateways. Human birth is a highly risky affair, with somewhere between one in four and one in three pregnancies ending in either miscarriage or stillbirth. For every successful fertilization of an egg, there exists the possibility of miscarriage, the possibility this new life may never become a fully formed fetus, a year-old baby, or a grown adult.

People who give birth are brave souls ~ brave warriors. Birthing a baby forces us to confront the inevitability of death. One day, this child we are bearing will die. If we are fortunate, that child will help us to die when we are old, and we won't have to watch him or her die. A friend told me that upon giving birth, she immediately became aware of how much she had to lose. By daring to give birth we dare to love, and to lose what we love. Watching one's child die is probably the most painful death one can experience.

My own sister lost a baby at birth, when her first child was born with an apparent heart defect. This brought the traumatic death of a child painfully close to home. When I arrived from out of town the day after the baby had died, my sister wanted me to hold her baby. Because I could see how much it meant to her, I agreed. The social worker brought the body of baby Devon wrapped in a blanket, cold from the refrigerator where her body was being stored before cremation. I held her in my arms and stared down at her perfect skin, tightly closed eyes, and thick strands of red hair. "How could she be so well formed, and yet not alive?" my mind wondered. Her death was hard to grasp. But the cold, still body, not breathing, made it very clear that her true being was elsewhere.

My whole family (but especially my mother) supported my sister in her grief journey over many years. We all experienced our own grief for the loss of this baby in our own way as well. I still feel angel spirit Devon with me at various points in my life.

In going through labor and delivery also, the woman herself enters a treacherous passageway. Several women have told me that in the worst moments of their labor, they wondered if they would actually make it through. Some women don't.[75] And many of those who would like to become pregnant find themselves unable to. Infertility is a surprisingly common experience, with over 15% of couples struggling to conceive. Infertility is a hidden form of loss that can cause as much strain and stress as facing cancer.[76] And while just as many cases of infertility are due to a factor in the male partner as in the female, the woman usually bears the brunt of public opinion. Most people worldwide believe that infertility is due primarily to the woman, causing shame and stigma, especially for women who are unable to bear children in poorer countries and may have little access to treatment.

Pregnancy loss and miscarriage can cause a woman to doubt her body. Mind-Body Coach for Women Esther Wyss-Flamm shares how Yoga helped her to reconnect inwardly after four miscarriages:

> *I had four miscarriages prior to adopting our daughter.*
> *Two years later I became a biological mom unexpectedly. I*
> *remember feeling deeply betrayed by my body, unbearably*

---

75. Although maternal mortality is low in most countries, it is still high in some.

76. Alice D. Domar and Alice Lesch Kelly. *Conquering Infertility: Dr. Alice Domar's Mind/Body Guide to Enhancing Fertility and Coping with Infertility* (New York: Penguin Books, 2004).

betrayed. Sex became mechanical. I pushed my body to cooperate with a fertility treatment that was just not right for me. I also remember how good and how soothing it felt to get back on the mat and move my body again - even though I was reluctant at first. My body led me into the movements that I so needed, hip openers and more.

The Moon Salutation can help in healing after miscarriage or other pregnancy loss. This story of experiencing miscarriage comes from Yoga Teacher Carly Conatser:

It's hard being thirty-eight and watching everyone I know get successfully pregnant and birth their babies along with the next phase of their lives. To ease my mind I follow I Had A Miscarriage *on Instagram and I connect with other women in my community who I know have as well. We get together for coffee, hikes, and Yoga.*

In my own body I turn to the Moon Salutation, the practice that feels the most feminine and sacred to bring healing to my grieving heart. The Moon Salutation reconnects me with my body's own cycle and timing.

I remember when I first learned the Moon Salutation as part of my Yoga teacher training at Kripalu. It was the first time I experienced grace and ease in my Yoga postures or flow. There was something more natural about this flow as it circled me around on my mat and gave me the opportunity to connect with the space I was practicing in.

It also connected me to the people around me. Up until that point, I had always set my mat as close to the front of the room as possible, something that followed me from the academic experience of wanting to be at the head of the class, close to the front so that I wouldn't be distracted by everyone else.

Yet, in this lunar flow, I witness the beauty of movement and become part of something larger than myself. I'm not trying to narrow my experience or put on blinders to avoid seeing anyone else around me. In flowing this way, I embody the experience that we all move in a circle, sometimes we're at the front, sometimes the back, and sometimes the middle. In life, we all take turns.

By nature, I'm a striver, and this practice has helped me tune in more to allowing freedom and natural rhythms to take the place of ambition, effort, and expectation. I become part of my own cycle with its waxing and waning moments. I realize that nothing has the power to separate me from my true self unless I give it the power to do so. Just like the moon, I can be present in my own darkness and not feel my light diminish.

▶   ▶   ▶

People of color, veterans, those with cancer, and transgender people experience higher than average rates of infertility, adding to the challenges they already face. African-American women experience not only a higher rate of infertility but also higher rates of infant prematurity, infant mortality, and maternal mortality than their white sisters. Even when comparing women of similar socio-economic status and levels of education, African-American women still have worse birth outcomes.[77] The exorbitant cost of many fertility treatments, and the fact that they are not covered by most health-insurance plans, put them out of the reach of many in the United States, let alone in the Global South.

We have a long way to go to face and reverse the lingering effects of racism and white supremacy that continue to permeate every aspect of our culture, including birth outcomes. We need to increase access to reproductive and infertility care for all women, all over the world, and also reproductive justice, whereby all people ~ no matter their race, ethnicity, country of origin, or socio-economic status ~ have the right and the ability to make healthy choices for themselves and their families.

---

77. Personal interview, Arisika Razak, June 21, 2019. Arisika attributes these differential birth outcomes to racism, and researchers now agree.

20

GROWING EVER MORE
COMPASSIONATE IN MENOPAUSE

Just as menarche is an initiation into the time of childbearing, so menopause is an initiation into a time *beyond* childbearing. Whether a woman has had children in her lifetime or not, this initiation still applies.

The fertile years are a constantly changing mix of hormones, with resulting physical and emotional fluctuations, all overlaid with the actual big events of this time of life - dating, mating, childbearing (or not) and the demands of family and career. Freed from the monthly hormonal swirl and from actual child-bearing, a post-menopausal woman is more available now to herself and to the world. Released from looking out for just her own child, she is available to turn her attention to all children, all humanity.

I worked with a spiritual teacher as I entered menopause, and one of the assignments she gave me was to read *The Awakening of Universal Motherhood*, by Sri Mata Amritanandamayi Devi, also known as Ammachi. Ammachi is a self-awakened teacher from South India, and the text I was assigned to read is a speech she gave when being granted the Gandhi-King Award for Non-Violence.

Awakened motherhood is love and compassion felt not only towards one's own children, but towards all people, animals and plants, rocks and rivers - a love extended to all of nature, all beings. Indeed, to a woman in whom the state of true motherhood has awakened, all creatures are

*her children. This love, this motherhood, is Divine Love –
and that is God.*[78]

Ammachi's comments are relevant to the opportunity we are
given at menopause. Menopause invites us to see not just our
own children but all of humanity's children, all our neighbors,
all sisters and brothers everywhere, as our children.[79]

Technically, menopause is the time when the menstrual cycle
ends. It is defined as the 12th month after a woman's last period
(or 24th month in the United Kingdom). Perimenopause is the
transition time of 5 to 15 years before actual menopause. During
perimenopause a woman's hormonal cascade bounces around like
an irregular Ferris wheel, not sure whether to start or stop or keep
going after all. Estrogen, progesterone, follicle stimulating hormone (FSH), luteinizing hormone (LH), and pituitary hormones
all fluctuate wildly, which can create havoc in the body and mind.

The passageway into menopause is narrow and hormonal
changes are massive. The brain must rewire itself to respond
to significantly lower hormone levels. The body must adjust to
changing signals from the brain and circulating hormones. The
adrenal glands must take up some of the slack as the ovaries
reduce their function, coming into rest. These changes are not
minor, as all hormones have emotional as well as physical effects,
controlling mood, sleep, sexual function, and so much more.

For many women, menopause is a crazy-wisdom initiation.
The surprising and sudden unpredictability of bleeding, hot
flashes, sleep, and emotions is incredibly disorienting. As challenging as monthly periods and emotions could be, there was
something comforting in knowing what to expect. Predictability
is wiped away in peri-menopause, and one must surrender totally

---

78. Sri Mata Amritanandamayi Devi (also known as Amma). *The Awakening
    of Universal Motherhood: Geneva Speech.* 2nd ed. (Kerala, India: Mata
    Amritanandamayi Mission Trust, 2004), 44.

79. My own mother became more empowered and open, more radiant and
    free beginning in her 50s. She became willing to stand up to my father,
    and grew out of the depression I had known her to exist in when I was a
    child. The change was so dramatic I sometimes barely recognized her. This
    woman who was so available to me emotionally, and who I consciously
    chose to embrace as an adult, was so different from the woman of my
    childhood memory.

or lose one's mind. For many women at this time sleep becomes difficult, as both estrogen and progesterone regulate sleep, and the body needs to find new pathways to deep rest.

As might be expected, waking regularly and repeatedly in the middle of the night can make one feel more than a little bit crazy. I needed to learn a new pace at menopause, resting more, ending my work day earlier, and relaxing more with fun movies, books, or sister companionship at night. Whereas before I had taken an intensive day or two off around my period for resting on the couch like a queen, I learned to spread that queen-dom out all month.

I noticed that when I rested sufficiently, my hot flashes went away. I also began to meditate, finding that it stabilized and calmed my entire being, something I desperately needed at this time.[80]

Menopause is rare in the animal kingdom. The vast majority of animal species remain fertile until death. Only two small species of whales, the orcas and small-finned pilot whales, go through a similar process. While childbearing takes a heavy toll on a woman's body especially as she ages and while infant survival rates go down in older mammals, the real evolutionary purpose for menopause lies in its social benefits. Women freed from childbearing begin to care for their children's children.[81] Older female orcas become a support to their pod, and especially in times of crisis such as low food supply, they serve as "repositories of ecological wisdom," such as where to find the scant salmon.[82]

While older women and men lose actual brain cells and some brain functions do decline with age, many other brain functions such as wise decision-making and emotional intelligence remain

---

80. I currently practice Heartfulness Meditation, a simplified form of Raja Yoga which focuses awareness on the heart. See www.Heartfulness.org for more information, and for referral to free trainers who can help you start meditating.

81. Ed Yong, "Why Killer Whales Go Through Menopause But Elephants Don't." *National Geographic.* March 5, 2015. https://www.nationalgeographic.com/science/phenomena/2015/03/05/why-killer-whales-go-through-menopause-but-elephants-dont/ (accessed January 17, 2019).

82. Ibid.

steady or even improve with age.[83] As much as our culture may disregard and dishonor aging, we need our elders to guide and support us. They play an invaluable, essential role in creating healthy families and communities.

As younger women, we need our post-menopausal sisters to help us grow into the best of who we are. Some of the best spiritual teachers I've known were everyday women in menopause. They exhibited a brilliance, generosity, and independence I've not seen in younger women.

A post-menopausal woman embodies all phases of the moon. She is aware of her own approaching death, and also the death of those around her. In this sense she embodies the dark half of the moon, the waning moon, the crone phase. But hormonally she is independent and free as she was as a girl, open to new creativity, new contributions. This is the waxing, new moon phase. A post-menopausal woman contains the blood mysteries within. A woman now holds all the phases of the moon in her body. Here is how Yoga Instructor Kendra West puts it:

My blood cycle used to remind me every month of the creatrix force I carried. As I've changed with age, I've become more like the new moon. These blood mysteries aren't lost but hidden in my body for a new phase of power. I reflect on the many faces of my goddess energy. The silver in my hair signifies that the ever-changing nature of blood and wisdom are within.

When I think of menopause I am reminded of Smashan Kali, the dark Goddess of Hinduism who dances on the cremation grounds. Kali embraces death as a great spiritual teacher. She does not grieve as she dances. She is totally free, enjoying herself with wild abandon. And although she has borne no children, she is known as the compassionate mother to all humanity.

---

83. Thomas Oxman, "Reflections on Aging and Wisdom." *The American Journal of Geriatric Psychiatry* 26, no. 11 (November, 2018). 1108-1118. See also Rettner, Rachael. "Why Older Adults Are "Happier." Live Science. May 29, 2013. https://www.livescience.com/34825-older-adults-happiness-negative-emotions (accessed May 13, 2019).

Kali's heart holds the worst of what life can be. She holds our worst moments and fears, and still says "It's okay." We can become like the model of Kali, wild and free, understanding that loss, just like the dark moon, cleans us out to receive what is new. Facing death reminds us that everything is temporary. It reminds us that life is a gift. It teaches us to love each moment and each person. Menopause brings us face-to-face with our own greatest fear ~ death ~ and thus frees us into the second half of our lives.

A woman's ability to surf the waves of her life is tested at menopause, and if she is successful in learning the lessons of this time, she will be forever a better surfer. She will surf not only her own waves of emotion and changing circumstances but be helpful to her sisters, daughters, and granddaughters as they, too, traverse the difficult passages of their lives.

Be gentle with yourself at this time. Take whatever space and time you need. Get extra support to figure out the changes you are going through. Despite how disorienting the transition can be, you are not crazy. This is a normal passage for women. Work with a good doctor, therapist, acupuncturist, chiropractor, Ayurvedic practitioner, or naturopath if need be. The body gradually adjusts to lower levels of hormones, and for most women, peace ultimately returns.

Anything in your life that has not been faced will need to be addressed. Give yourself time to find your bearings. Experiment with what will make you truly happy. You may need to make some big shifts ~ career changes, location changes, relationship changes. You may need to change your bedtime or other sleeping arrangements. You may just need to get out and have more fun, join a new club, take up a new sport, or make new friends. Especially at menopause, a women's circle can provide a wonderful support.

Women in menopause often experience days of high energy and days of very little or no energy. During menopause, you will have to gauge your energy on different days. Sometimes the Moon Salutation may be perfect; sometimes floor poses and restorative poses will be in order.

On days when you are feeling exhausted or haven't slept the night before, restorative poses are invaluable, and will steady the mind and body, preparing you to face the day ahead. Restorative poses in the late afternoon or evening help with sleep the following evening. Practice the poses in Chapter 16 or even better, get yourself to a good restorative Yoga class and receive the total nurturance of the teacher. On days when you have more energy, get aerobic exercise or follow your body as to what would be helpful. Practice the Moon Salutation to maintain strength and flexibility and to steady your nervous system with its deep breathing and steady flow.

Yoga in post-menopause keeps the legs and spine strong, helping to prevent falls and maintain bone health. It supports flexibility and overall suppleness, heart health, happiness, and a strong immune system. Keep doing your Yoga as you age, even as you add new fun activities into your life!

I love the Moon Salutation now that I am post-menopausal, because it helps me stay juicy and creative, alive in my hips. During my worst peri-menopausal days, restorative Yoga was what saved me, but now I'm ready for standing and flowing again. Many women experience sexual dryness in menopause, but I find that flowing in and out of the squats as well as Lunge and Triangle Poses brings circulation to the yoni in a way that almost nothing else does. I love being juicy and alive in all chakras, all vital parts of my body.

PART FIVE: HEALING, POWER, AND PEACE

21

LOVING OUR BODIES ~ WOMEN'S SELF-IMAGE

How could anyone ever tell you
You were anything less than beautiful?
How could anyone ever tell you
You were less than whole?
How could anyone fail to notice
That your loving is a miracle?
How deeply you're connected to my soul.

~ Libby Roderick[84]

I love my body as I love the earth.

~ Sign I made and posted in my office.

As women enter the healing process, we often make a conscious choice to love ourselves despite the negative body image so many of us have internalized. We may practice loving self-affirmations, or simply attempt to interrupt self-criticism each time we notice it. I have been amazed at the tenacity of this problem even among women desiring to heal and change. No matter what, it seems as though we can always find something wrong with our bodies.

---

84. Libby Roderick, "How Could Anyone Ever Tell You." If You See a Dream. Anchorage, Alaska: Turtle Island Records (1990), compact disc.

The Moon Salutation is a tremendous help in this regard. It instills an internal sense of dignity, something which grows spontaneously through the practice of Yoga poses, but which is accentuated for women in the flowing movements of the Moon Salutation. The emphasis on belly, the rounded shape of the arms as they move in and out of Temple Pose, and the curvaceousness of the Moon Salutation overall help us honor the rounded fullness of women, a natural form that is devalued by our culture.

The Moon Salutation awakens the inner experience of grace and strength, replacing self-criticism with acceptance. Elizabeth Shillington, a practitioner of the Moon Salutation, describes how her self-image softens and expands to include the earth body when practicing this flow. "I'm not in a judgmental mode about how well or poorly I do the movements, but in a peaceful state of attunement with the earth and an acceptance of my body as part of her."

I will often invite women to use the practice of the Moon Salutation as a way to enter into a gentler relationship with their bodies. If they are unable to hold a sense of love for themselves, I invite them to at least hold it for another ~ to see the partner they may be mirroring or the group as a whole with loving eyes.

From my Journal in 1997: YMCA Moon Yoga Class

The theme of today's class is women's body image. I ask participants to take a few minutes to contemplate their relationship to their bodies. I ask them to pay attention to any reactions that may have come up when I said, "women's body image," such as "Oh, shit."

We consider various parts of the body one by one ~ feet, knees, hips, belly, uterus (or space where it would be if it had not been surgically removed such as via hysterectomy), yoni (birth passage and vulva), ribs, lungs, breasts, shoulders, neck, and head.

We then slide back through time, reflecting on the ways we have worked with our body image over time, different perspectives we have taken to find ways to love ourselves completely.

I allow time for journaling, and then invite the women to share. Listening to these women, I realize that the two areas most often mentioned for dislike are belly and breasts, the areas that most clearly define us as women. I feel sad about the pain that is shared. Shame over starting menstruation early or late. Dislike for one's breasts, pain that the breasts and hips never filled out or that they are too big, wishing the tummy were flatter, fighting with the body to keep it in shape and worry that having children will make that battle impossible.

I am moved by their honesty. I invite the group to take a deep breath. I suggest that we hold space for each other to move and grow from these places, that just because a woman has shared dislike of her body does not mean she will always feel it.

I tell them we are going to practice the Moon Salutation together now as a way to feel a positive relationship to our bodies. I encourage them to feel the stability of the breath, and to experience compassion and love for themselves exactly as they are. I invite them to feel their flowing strength, their power and energy. One woman shares that she feels weak and awkward in the squatting poses because they are hard for her.

Ordinarily we don't use the mirror, but today I invite them to turn toward it. I ask them to fuzz up their eyes so that they see their reflections not as individuals, but instead as many manifestations of the Goddess. We begin to enter the flow.

I suggest we visualize ourselves in a natural setting, such as a grassy hill overlooking a pond. "Are there animals?" I ask. "Yes, deer are grazing around us," answers one woman. "And the full moon is rising directly in front of us," says another. And so we begin.

When we complete I have them turn to a partner and mirror each other through the flow. "If you have trouble feeling yourself as the Goddess, at least feel it for the woman you are looking at," I say. As we complete, I invite them to feel compassion and love for themselves. As they leave the session, I encourage them to carry some of this self-love with them, even a little bit.

22

THE TRANSFORMATIVE
POWER OF A CIRCLE

In a circle, participants face in to a common center, sometimes marked by a candle, sometimes marked by nothing at all. Circles create a sense of being held in this life together. They remind us of our shared journey as women and of our place in the greater web of humanity. They remind us that we are not alone as we face the challenges of our lives.

With their lateral orientation, Moon Salutations invite relatedness and connection to others. They are perfectly suited to practicing in a circle or facing a partner. When in a circle, the particular quality of each movement is enhanced by the collective strength of the group. The side-bending movements of Crescent Moon gain fluidity in a circle, the squats feel powerfully earthy and rooted, and the inspiration of Triangle Pose is made even brighter.

I will often have women look around at the group as we come into Goddess Pose. I might ask them what qualities they see. Women call out what they see ~ strength, power, love, and more. They then recognize that they are part of the whole that has generated those qualities. We are looking at each other as if looking at a circle of Goddesses.

Many teachers told me how the Moon Salutation itself calls them to practice in a circle, where they as teacher aren't standing out in front. Says Megha Nancy Buttenheim, co-creator of the Moon Salutation, "Often in Yoga class we're doing everything straight ahead. But I never like to lead the Moon Salutation as 'Hey everybody, look at me.' I lead it in a circle. It's a collective.

We look at one another as women do." This flow by its very nature helps women to bond. As Yoga retreat leader Tracie Sage said, "Sisterhood is very strong in those classes, definitely."

Deva Parnell, Moon Salutation Co-Creator, shared how she loves to watch the circle turn with multiple repetitions of the Moon Salutation, and how this helps to connect the group:

The Moon Salutation is a circle of postures and also a circle of women.

We step to the right every time and I end up back at the beginning where I started – the wheel turns. This flow reminds us that we're not alone. We don't live in a vacuum. Communication and connection between women is so important.

Combining sharing circles with Yoga practice or other sacred movement can deepen the healing effect. The circle of the group creates a womb-like wholeness for holding powerful experience of the group and individuals in it. Kripalu Yoga Teacher Deborah Foss describes the liberating effects of sharing our vulnerabilities and wounds:

Women find power in claiming ourselves, in sharing our wounds. We own where we are and where we've been. We share commonalities and differences, our uniqueness, our bodies, marital status, children or childlessness, our abuse history, mental health history. It's a challenge to acknowledge that we have been raped or incested, yet still see each other as whole. If anything, women become more loving as these stories are shared. Sharing in a circle like this is liberating. We realize that our soul is more important than our experience. The soul transcends body, experience, age, shape.

Circles connect women in supporting each other's growth. As women come to know each other in the circle, they begin to root for their sisters, inwardly cheering for the woman across the room and releasing self-criticism in the process.

Circles can also support cross-generational ties. They help us understand each other better and deepen our compassion for all phases of women's lives, phases we either have or will go through. An early resident of Kripalu who preferred to remain anonymous told me about the cross-generational sharing in the Women and Yoga program:

> *One of the most powerful things we did was to have the participants talk about all levels of womanhood. Young women talked about menstruation and becoming sexual. Other women would talk about motherhood. And the crones shared about aging. Hearing the wisdom of each age was so moving. Especially the older women. They talked about what it was like to lose their attractiveness. Often they lost their husbands, their children. All of the women gained a lot of power from that cross-generational sharing.*

The bonding encouraged by the Moon Salutation and women's circles in general stands in opposition to the isolation many women experience in the rest of their lives. Says Deborah Foss, "Our culture does not foster sisterhood or even community at all. We are the culture of the rugged individualist, the I-can-do-it culture, the I-can-be-better culture. It is not about 'we.' We are isolated in our I-ness." The Moon Salutation helps to reduce this isolation.

As healing and powerful as circles are, they are not always that way, and not for all women at all times. Every one of us is sensitive to inclusion/exclusion. Women can feel left out because of ethnicity, color, size, age, perceived ability or non-ability, sexual expression, gender expression, socio-economic status, education, country of origin, language, and so much more. Even where women appear the same some may not feel comfortable. On the other hand, women who appear to be very different may actually be completely at ease, even when they are the only one with an obvious difference in a group.

Each woman makes choices about which circles are or might not be right for her. At the same time, skillful leadership can expand the range of who will feel truly welcome in a given group. This is why I am so passionate about teaching women's leadership skills, making more and more empowering circles available to more and more women.

▶   ▶   ▶

In India, most temples are created in a roughly rectangular design. The only temples created in a circle are Goddess temples from Northeastern India, temples dedicated to the Divine Mother in her many forms. Statues of various forms of the Goddess face inward in these temples, as if a circle of Divine Women were sharing sacred space together.

Could it be that this reflects an aspect of women's psychology, biology, and even spirituality? That at our best we see each other as sisters, as equals, and that not just our physical and emotional health but also our spiritual growth are enhanced by consciously joining together in sisterhood, as in a circle?

In my experience, a sacred circle of women creates a powerful vortex, an alchemy of love, wherein anything that needs to be released is melted away, anything that needs to be transformed is made whole. The power of such a circle magnifies the energy of the heart chakra, radiating love to each group member. A flavor of tenderness permeates the circle, and those who are open to it will find it seeping into every cell, touching and tumbling the heart into even more love.

I have often returned home after such a circle so profoundly radiant that my husband could not help but comment. A women's circle may not lead to actual bodily orgasm, but the turn-on of love is palpable, leading to profound and lasting healing. We inhale love, we exhale love. It is intoxicating. After practicing the Moon Salutation and being together in a circle, women remember this experience. We take it home with us as a precious memory, a treasured gift, enhancing and enlivening our continued Yoga practice.

YOGA FOR INCARCERATED TEEN GIRLS

Mary Lynn Fitton, RN, directs the Art of Yoga Project, a non-profit organization that brings Yoga and creative arts to incarcerated teen girls. Mary Lynn learned the Moon Salutation 20 years ago from an early version of this book and immediately began to integrate it into her curriculum.

Here is Mary Lynn's story:

The dimly lit room is cold and cinder blocked. Three pro-bation staff members chat loudly about their weekend at a high narrow desk.

We sit in a circle of 12 teenaged girls who wiggle and fidget on their purple yoga mats. I think to myself how young a few girls look and my heart breaks a little.

"There's not much good about being a girl," remarks Trayna. *We have already gone around the circle sharing our names and the pros and cons of womanhood at our check-in. The girls here, ages 12-17, come from underserved and under-resourced communities. In the gang culture many of them come from, men have all the power. Some of the girls have been sex trafficked; most have been sexually abused; all have experienced trauma. To guide them toward self-love and self-respect is a tall order. But we are up for it.*

Today my co-teacher, Shikha, reads from our Yoga and Creative Arts Curriculum to the girls:

"The Sun Salutations are an expression of the male. Think of the sun ... fire, heat, lots of energy is required for all of those push-ups. The Moon Salutation, in contrast, is more fluid. It honors the cycles of the moon and our cycles as women. It is circular and includes mostly movement to the side. The Moon Salutation also brings us into the feminine principle of receiving with many poses that open our arms wide to all that life has to offer."

Later in the practice, the girls will write in journals to prompts like:

My body has the power to ...

A woman's body is unique because ...

My cycle as a woman represents my abilities to ...

Feminine qualities that anyone, male or female or gender-non conforming, could express are ...

To me, feeling feminine feels like ...

Afterward, in their check-out, they will share about women they admire and give blessings to themselves and each other.

But for now, it's time to move.

The girls know the Moon Salutation well and Isha asks if she can lead today. For seven beautiful minutes, a calm comes over Unit 5. We flow. We breathe. Rayn says, "This feels hella good." We listen to Isha using her "Yoga teacher voice" and Shikha and I share a smile.

Why Women Need Sisterhood

Amazingly, women were eliminated from the vast majority of more than 60 years of research on stress because our hormonal cycles were thought to complicate the stress response. Researchers felt they could get a clearer, more accurate picture of the stress response by studying men only. [85]

For this reason, the very different response of women to stress was overlooked and obscured. The standard explanation of stress as "fight or flight" was said to apply equally to both sexes. Instead, when women actually were studied researchers found that women have a very different stress response of a strong need for affiliation. Instead of "fight or flight," a group of researchers at UCLA found that the female response to stress is better characterized as "tend and befriend." As Shelley Taylor, lead researcher in the study wrote:

Women's responses to stress are characterized by patterns that involve caring for offspring under stressful circumstances, joining social groups to reduce vulnerability, and contributing to the development of social groupings, especially those involving female networks, for the exchange of resources and responsibilities.[86]

More than 30 different studies have found that while men tend to isolate during stress, women instead turn to others, activating their social networks. This is one of the most reliable, robust sex differences that exists. [87] In conditions of high stress, such as poverty, illness, extreme heat, overcrowding, being placed in a new environment, or even waiting to take a test, women will seek affiliation with others - preferentially other women - to calm and soothe them.[88]

---

85. Shelley E. Taylor et. al. "Biobehavioral Responses to Stress in Females: Tend-and-Befriend, Not Fight-or-Flight." *Psychological Review* 107, No. 3 (2000). 411-429.

86. Ibid, 421-422.

87. Ibid, 422.

88. Shelley E. Taylor, *The Tending Instinc : How Nurturing is Essential for Who We Are and How We Live* (New York: USA Macmillan, 2002), ebook, Chapter 6: Women Befriending.

And this social connection is good for women's health. Female friendships are profoundly positive. A Stanford study of women with terminal breast cancer found that those who were placed in support groups lived twice as long, or a year and a half longer, than women not placed in support groups.[89] A Harvard Medical School study of more than 12,000 nurses showed that women with stronger female networks were happier and less likely to become ill as they aged. According to the Harvard study, not having a close friend was as significant a health risk for women as smoking or being severely overweight.[90]

The central hormone that likely explains the tendency toward "tend and befriend" in women is oxytocin, released by both men and women during times of stress. Oxytocin is responsible for bonding, for creating the desire to protect children and join with others in a communal way. It is released in large amounts during childbirth, nursing, and sex, but also in positive social interactions such as hugging, massage, and even greeting friends. The effects of oxytocin are accentuated by estrogen, but inhibited by testosterone, explaining the different effects it may have on men and women during stress.[91]

All of the advice we had been giving to women about stress ‒ go to the gym and exercise, take a walk outside and get some fresh air, do Yoga and breathe ‒ was only partially correct. We should have included as the number one stress buster for women: find other women and connect. Create a network of confidantes you can trust. Build friendships and maintain them over time.

Many women have been conditioned by our culture to consider other women as threats or competitors. Healing any sense of competition is key for women. When our sisters thrive, we all thrive, and when we build loyal, supportive friendships with an ever-widening circle, our well-being is enhanced. Sharing with women is good not just for creating a feeling of interconnectedness and belonging, but on a very literal level for reducing stress hormones in our bodies. So go practice your Yoga with a friend! And find a women's circle. It's good for your health.

89. Taylor, *The Tending Instinct,* ebook, Chapter 5: A Little Help from Friends and Strangers.

90. Jacqueline Mroz, *Girl Talk: What Science Can Teach Us About Female Friendship* (New York: Seal Press, 2018), 204.

91. Taylor et al. "Biobehavioral Responses to Stress in Females," 416.

23

RECOVERING FROM TRAUMA
AND SEXUAL ABUSE

No matter how much a woman has been stamped down,
her inner flame still remains, even if only as a small ember.
What fans the flame is growing the Inner Mother.

~ Clarisa Pinkola Estes, author,
Women Who Run with the Wolves

For many reasons this chapter has been the most challenging for me to write. I have personally experienced trauma and abuse. I know well the pain that is suffered in this healing process. It lies deep in my bones and in every cell of my being. And yet I struggle to find the words to do it justice. I wonder if I even need to clarify what is meant by violence against women: the continuing relevance of the #MeToo movement, the ongoing revelations of sexual abuse by spiritual teachers (including by Kripalu Yoga's Founder, Amrit Desai), the alarmingly high percentage of women who have been raped or were molested as children; the devaluation of our mothers and of mothering; the rape and pillage of our first mother and essential ground of being, the earth; the loss of women's traditions through the burning of the witches in Europe and America and the suppression of women's spiritual experience in India. We all know these things, and still the voices inside me wonder ~ am I making it up? Maybe it really isn't all that bad . . . .

What happens when women who have been for centuries ~ no, millennia ~ devalued, ignored, shamed, and raped enter an embodied practice which is at its core life-affirming, loving, empowering, and totally honoring of their female being? What happens when women who have been sexually abused, or simply told by prim grandmothers to keep their knees together, join with a sacred circle of women and there enter powerful hip-opening postures: Five-Pointed Star, Triangle, Goddess, and Full Squat? When women share in the embodied practice of Yoga with the intention to support each other in re-honoring our female selves, the results are unspeakably profound.

You don't need to have specifically experienced abuse in order to carry its effects in your body. Trauma is so widespread in our society that it touches every one of us, especially as women. Trauma is passed down from generation to generation and often reactivated in painful, fresh experiences in this lifetime.

But this book is not about the losses or the violence. It is about healing. It is about the courage and vulnerability needed to reclaim our essential purity and integrity, our beauty and our strength.

At the first Women and Yoga program held at the Kripalu Center in November of 1988, it soon became apparent that it was not possible to celebrate the female body without also opening to the pain held there for so long. This program combined Yoga postures with what Kripalu calls "Self Discovery," a blend of inner exploration, spiritual practice, and group support and sharing. Megha Nancy Buttenheim, co-director of that first program in which 80 women participated, spoke of it as "planetary" and "gorgeous," saying later that she wasn't in as powerful a program again for 10 years.

Deva Parnell, an assistant in the program, elaborated on the surprising intensity of the week:

> *The Women and Yoga program at Kripalu opened up the whole idea of exploring the nature of the feminine and the feminine experience of Yoga as being different from the male. . . It was like opening up Pandora's box. We had no idea of the things it was going to ignite, such as the anger*

that came out as women were given room to explore femi-
nine issues and at the same time to do Yoga, an embodied
practice that accesses old memories.

The opening to embodiment and sexuality represented in the
Moon Salutation reflects the wider cultural exploration of these
areas at the time. As Jungian psychologist Marion Woodman
points out, bringing sexuality to consciousness has been a dominant concern of our age, making it impossible to hide the existence
of sexual violence and its devastating consequences. Previously
these had existed as part of the collective shadow.[92]

In Yogic practice, sexual repression has been an unfortunate
consequence of the misunderstanding of ancient teachings regarding sexuality. The intent of these teachings was not to repress
sexuality but instead to cultivate a mind and being which would
be peaceful enough for spiritual practice. Unfortunately, where
sexual energy is not owned and integrated in a healthy way, it
becomes relegated to the shadow of the personality, where it is
frequently harmful to oneself or to others.

Rather than requiring or elevating purity, the Moon Salutation
opens us to embodiment and sexuality. By opening the hips in
the context of this beautiful flowing sequence, the split is healed
between what was allowed and what was disallowed, between
purity and sexuality, between virgin and whore. In recognizing
the physical need of women to strengthen and relax the pelvis,
sexual issues are no longer hidden but are brought to the surface.
The creators of the Moon Salutation inadvertently, but perhaps
necessarily, touched this powerful current in American culture.

Here is Tracie Sage speaking about the way Yoga and the
Moon Salutation helped her to open where she had been injured:

After recovering from sexual abuse I noticed how the Moon
Salutation opens the pelvis. I hadn't even been aware how
much I was tensing in my stomach and in my vagina.
Practicing the Moon Salutation showed me that and also
helped me to release the tension. It's hard to say which came
first - healing from sexual abuse or my Yoga practice. They

---

92. Woodman, Marion. *Addiction to Perfection: The Still Unravished Bride*
(Toronto: Inner City Books, 1982).

supported each other. Now when I practice the Moon Salutation I notice that I'm very open there.

In disregarding our boundaries, our abusers violated the integrity of our chakras, especially the lower chakras. The Moon Salutation helps us to recover that integrity.

Whether or not we have personally experienced sexual violence, many people are not comfortable feeling their pelvis and yoni; they would prefer to remain disconnected, as our culture prefers. Valerie Kit Love, occupational therapist and Yoga teacher, talks about this aspect of the Moon Salutation:

The Moon Salutation in particular opens the inner thighs and is aligned to the lower chakras. The low belly and back, groin, and buttocks are where safety, creativity, sexuality, and receptivity are held. Most of us have unfinished business regarding these issues and hold unconscious tension in this part of the body. We walk around protecting it. The most vulnerable part of ourselves has to open in the Moon Salutation and not many people like that.

According to psychologist Marion Woodman, the foundation of a woman's healing is recovering her own felt body sense, for in this way she repairs the broken connection to her own being. Yoga is a tremendous help in this regard, as it allows one to access the physical body and through it, one's authentic feelings.

Kripalu Yoga teacher Deborah Foss explains this process:

When we're in our heads, concepts get frozen. Often when emotions come up we don't know what to do with them. That's why I love integrating self-discovery and Yoga ~ they complement each other so beautifully. Yoga helps us to shift gears and keep things moving. It allows the energy to transform.

Making a conscious choice to reconnect with the body is an important step in giving birth to one's true self. As Woodman states, a woman's "only real hope is to care for her own body and experience it as the vessel through which her Self may be born."[93]

---

93. Woodman, 1980, 100.

While for many women it has been unsafe to be present in the body, the practice of Yoga allows one to be with the body in a way that is safe and comfortable.

While Yoga in general is beneficial for accessing the felt body sense, the Moon Salutation is especially helpful for women who have chosen to enter this healing process. It not only opens us to our bodies, but does so in a context that explicitly honors our female being. It allows women to feel both our strength and our beauty. And it enacts the postures that have been most prohibited to women. As women especially, we were not given permission to spread our legs wide and to feel the power of that stance. As women practice the Moon Salutation we are partaking in a radical act of self-empowerment and love.

As women come into the squat in the company of other women, we open to our vulnerability in a way that is at the same time completely safe. Again, Deborah Foss observes how liberating this is: "The squat is about giving birth to yourself as a woman. In this culture it's not really safe to keep your knees apart and here is a place to let go of all of that pent-up tension in a group that's safe and supportive. It's so liberating." We find that a new sense of our soul can emerge as we let go of old injuries and open the places where the hurt has been held.

Yoga Teacher Carly Conatser writes how healing the Moon Salutation is for both her and her students:

The Moon Salutation was my go-to sequence when I taught Yoga for healing from sexual trauma in New York City nonprofits and studios. Eight years later in Kentucky, it's what I offer when I teach workshops for college students impacted by sexual violence. Often, my students will echo what I feel, that the Moon Salutation helps them be strong, feminine, and integrated within a community. "Moving this way made me feel less alone," wrote one of my students.

When I step on my mat and flow, I find wholeness within. I nourish my body in a way that feels attuned to who I am as a woman. In my miscarriage and being sexually assaulted, my body experienced shame. In the Moon Salutation I give my body back what it lost.

It takes courage and vulnerability to reclaim our essential purity and integrity. The Moon Salutation takes women to the deep place of honesty and openness needed to effect healing, and turns on its head the cultural devaluation of the feminine. It instills not just ordinary self-esteem and self-empowerment, but an understanding of oneself as a truly sacred aspect of the divine.

MY EXPERIENCE OF ABUSE AND HEALING

A warning as we continue ~ the next few paragraphs may be difficult to read. I pray that by including them I may give courage to women who have experienced their own trauma, although different from mine. This section also gives broader context to the role the Moon Salutation plays in my ongoing healing and wholeness. For those who would like more detail, I recommend you read the book chapter "#MeToo: How I Healed from Incest to Recover the Divine Feminine Within."[94] Here I will tell the story very briefly.

As a child I experienced physical, sexual, and emotional abuse. My parents were well intentioned but came from extremely repressive backgrounds. I was raised in Christian Science, a restrictive religion. We did not go to doctors or talk openly about the human body and its needs, let alone emotional or psychological needs.

As I grew, my father was sexually intrusive. When I was seven he secretly showed me his penis and asked if I'd like to touch. He talked to me about my period long before my mom had even mentioned it. When I was a teen he confided in me the challenges they were having in their sexual relationship and showed me the birth control they used. The only dream I remember from youth is of my father chasing me with a knife as I ran away from him on a burning boat.

Pausing, I breathe deeply as I write. This is hard to talk about… And I know I'm safe, and you're safe as you read it.

It never occurred to me to tell anyone. I was frozen inside and totally cut off from my feelings. Many years later in therapy I realized I had been terrified and profoundly distanced from

---

94. Cornell, Laura. "Me Too: How I Healed from Incest to Recover the Divine Feminine Within." In *The Game Changer (Volume 3): Inspirational Stories that Changed Lives*, edited by Iman Aghay, (Vancouver, Canada: Success Road Enterprises, 2018), 233-244.

my mother. In my late teens and early twenties I experienced an eating disorder, anxiety and depression, and finally chronic fatigue. Talk therapy improved my relationship with food but did little to address my spiraling emotions or the chronic fatigue.

I am incredibly grateful for the transformation I've experienced since those times, now almost 30 years ago. The journey home has been long. Everything already mentioned in this book - learning to love my body, honoring its wisdom, and circling with other women - was critical. Two foundational keys through all of this were healing my relationship with the inner feminine and discovering Yoga.

As Tracie said above, it's hard to tell which came first, finding Yoga or healing from sexual abuse. I consider Yoga an incredible gift without which my life would have taken a completely different, and much more negative, trajectory. Not only did my chronic fatigue resolve, but I learned to ground my emotions in my body. I began to honor my authentic feelings and sensations, a radical departure from my childhood. Yoga is what brought me home to myself, and what continues to do so, every time I practice. Sisterhood and Yoga combined have provided the container for me to gently but steadily reweave the web with my inner ground of being.

Sadly, I also believe I was abused by my uncle as a baby. In preparing to write this book, I asked myself the question, "What does my uncle's molestation of me have to do with this book?" Here is the answer that came:

From my Journal: August 18, 2018

This is an important part of my journey. My uncle hurt me, but he does not define me.

Molestation rips one away from the soul, from the core of who we are. Healing is a gradual process - every day coming back to the truth of the body and its goodness. The body is not stained, not impure, but our feelings can be warped, bent inside a psyche that does not know how to open. Yoga helps to reshape and open that psyche.

The beauty of the Moon Salutation is in learning to say "No." My legs in Goddess Squat are the feet of the baby wanting to push the abuser away, the strength of that push, that "No." This is why the Goddess squat is so needed by women. In trauma legs want to run, or for a baby, legs want to push away and kick. "Leave me alone!" they say. "I don't like that!" they say. "No!"

For a woman, living a full life comes from reclaiming her wholeness, and that means reclaiming, bringing home, all the parts of ourselves that were left behind in the trauma, all the parts that were frozen in confused fear, in confused overwhelm.

The Moon Salutation has the sideways gentleness of Crescent Moon Pose. This woman who has been damaged is going to be okay. She can heal. She can reclaim her fullness, herself. She is safe. I feel gentle, ready, and open.

Creating embodied safety in the Moon Salutation is similar to the "titration" recommended in somatic therapy. We don't dive 100% into the pain all at once, which can be over-stimulating and counterproductive. We go into it in little bits, small pieces, one at a time, knowing we are safe....

Goddess Squat ~ "No." I'm here, I'm powerful, and I'm not going to take it.

Triangle Pose ~ I'm not alone. Angels are watching over me. Angelic forces care for and protect me, no matter what.

Pyramid Pose ~ I can be quiet. I can sleep. Trauma can steal your peace. Nightmares, anxiety, and panic attacks, frequently lasting for decades, can rob one of the joy that is our birthright. I deserve rest. I am worthy of ease.

Lunge ~ I have a beautiful life in front of me. No one can steal my opportunity to live fully. I can choose the best path and move forward in ways that support my unique unfolding.

Side Lunge ~ The earth is my witness. The earth is protecting me, caring for me, guiding me. Just as the Buddha touched the earth when the demon was threatening him, and just as the Buddha asked Mother Earth to witness for him in that moment, so I touch the ground, calling for Mother Earth to companion me. Mother Earth is always with me. She supports me as I heal from this abuse.

Full Squat ~ I am stable, secure, whole. I am safe as I rest in simplicity and in my connection to the earth. Here is emptiness, birth, and also fullness. I feel the roots of my body opening down into the earth. My yoni is open, but I know I'm safe. Like a woman who is well-companioned in childbirth, I am well companioned in my Full Squat Pose.

Healing from trauma isn't easy. We need our sisters (and brothers) in this work. And we need Yoga flows like the Moon Salutation to remind us we are safe to feel, find, and reclaim our empowerment, our "no," our boundaries. Yoga helps the nervous system to heal. Rather than overwhelming us with extensive reminders of the trauma, Yoga allows us to experience them in small bits, integrating each wave of pain in digestible pieces.

For those of us healing from trauma or abuse of any kind, the moon is a helpful guide. With her many phases, she reminds us that everything flows in a circle. We go through confusion and pain, but the moon reminds us that the light will return, better times will come. The moon reminds us of our wholeness.

A woman who is recovering from sexual violence or abuse of any kind deserves the guidance of a trained psychotherapist. If you are recovering from incest, assault, harassment, or any other trauma, I recommend you work with a private counselor who can help you unravel your emotions and help you find your best path forward. Likewise, if you are using Yoga for recovery from trauma, please don't think that Yoga classes are a replacement for psychotherapy. They are a very needed adjunct, but not a replacement.

The Moon Salutation helps us to reconnect with our authentic body feeling and with each other, giving us the staying-power needed to effect our healing. As we feel the strength of our legs in the Moon Salutation, we are renewed, we know we are up for the healing journey that is required, and we are given courage by each other and by Mother Earth.

24

THE HEROINE'S JOURNEY OF DESCENT AND RETURN

Modern woman ... must make the journey into the dark regions below, and back again. She too, must experience the sacred mystery within her own body and revere it both as sacred and as a mystery.

~ Marion Woodman, *The Owl Was a Baker's Daughter: Obesity, Anorexia Nervosa and the Repressed Feminine*

As women we face joys and sorrows, times of challenge but also times of beauty and celebration. Traveling through difficult life experiences represents a dip into the dark. Whether a woman is healing from trauma and abuse or learning to love her body, which she may not have loved so well previously, whether she is weathering one of the rocky transitions of the female life cycle, resting on her period, or simply facing her own limitations and frailty ~ she is undertaking the journey of descent.

We all experience dipping into the dark, over and over again. Learning to face these dips with grace and humility is a big part of becoming whole. We return from facing the dark places in our lives renewed, ready to shine our light in the world. This journey of descent and ascent is seen also in the phases of the moon, which darkens completely and then returns to awe-inspiring fullness each month.

THE STORY OF INANNA ~ A MYTH OF DESCENT AND RETURN

The heroine's journey of descent and return is enacted in the myth of the Sumerian Great Goddess Inanna who descends to the underworld. Inanna's stories and poems were recorded on clay tablets dating to 2000 BCE along with striking illustrations.[95] Inanna's romance with her husband Dumuzi is the oldest love poem in the world. It long predates Hindu love tales from the *Puranas* such as Parvati with Shiva or Radha with Krishna as well as the *Song of Solomon* from the Hebrew scriptures.

In her many stories, Inanna is portrayed as Queen of Heaven and Earth, powerful and beautiful. As felt at the beginning of the Moon Salutation in the grandeur and breadth of the arms sweeping sideways from Mountain to Temple Pose, the stories of Inanna begin with her celebration. "When she leaned against the apple tree, her vulva was wondrous to behold. Rejoicing at her wondrous vulva, the young woman Inanna applauded herself."[96] Here is unabashed pride and joy in the female body, so different from the way many of us were raised.

Yet Inanna decides to leave her status and power in the above world to journey to the underworld:

From the Great Above the goddess opened her ear to the Great Below.
From the Great Above Inanna opened her ear to the Great Below.[97]

The Great Below represents the unconscious, the earth, the darkness, or the depths. The word for "ear" in Sumerian is the same as the word for "wisdom." In listening to the depths, Inanna was showing her desire for true wisdom.

The stated purpose of Inanna's journey is to visit her sister Ereshkigal, queen of the underworld, whose husband has died.

---

95. Wolkstein, Diane & Kramer, Samuel Noah. *Inanna: Queen of Heaven and Earth: Her Stories and Hymns from Sumer* (New York: Harper and Row, 1983).

96. Ibid, 12.

97. Ibid, 52.

In her descent Inanna must become completely naked. At each of seven gates she is stripped of one of her royal garments, jewels, or magical tools. Symbolically, in dipping into the dark we leave behind all that is familiar. Each new challenge forces us to confront the unknown, including our own unknown inner territory. As Inanna questions the removal of her clothes and jewelry, she is told, "Silence, Inanna. The ways of the underworld are perfect."[98] None of us enjoys the difficult life experiences we are given, and we fail to appreciate how necessary they are in our growth.

Inanna arrives "naked and bowed low" in front of her sister Ereshkigal, who condemns her to death. "Inanna was turned into a corpse ... and hung from a hook on the wall."[99] Why was Inanna condemned to death? Some say there is no reason, but that in deciding to tread where we have never been before, in choosing to enter the dark, we must lose everything on a spiritual level, including our previous understandings and coping mechanisms. What worked before will not work now, and we become as if dead to the world. In Yoga practice we experience this total surrender in the final pose of each session: *Shavasana* (corpse pose).

Inanna remains in the underworld, hanging from the hook for three full days. The three days of her death in this story mirror the three nights of the dark moon and the three primary days of a woman's bleeding, all times of rest and surrender. They also pre-date the famous story of Christ's three days in the tomb after the crucifixion. Poet and scholar of women's history Judy Grahn holds that the menstrual cycle and its correlation with lunar cycles formed the basis of early myths, including that of Inanna, and that these were later borrowed by religious traditions worldwide, such as in this case by Christianity.[100]

Inanna's companion Ninshubur has been holding watch in the above world, and when Inanna does not return, Ninshubur sends help to rescue her and bring her back to her position as Great Goddess. It is wise to have a witness if not a true companion on the journey. While Ninshubur did not descend with Inanna, she was standing by, ready to be of help when needed. Similarly,

---

98. Ibid, 58.

99. Ibid, 60.

100. Grahn, Judy. *Blood, Bread, and Roses: How Menstruation Created the World*, (Boston: Beacon Press, 1993), 212-214.

when we enter dangerous and unknown territory, it's a good idea to alert a friend, to tell our circle of sisters where we're going, or to have a therapist or mentor on call.

Like the moon, Inanna dies in order to be reborn. The Moon Salutation enacts the cycle of death and rebirth inherent in the cycles of nature: day and night, summer and winter, the light and dark phases of the moon. Embodying these cycles in our Yoga practice is a way of healing, embedding us in the larger context of life.

▶   ▶   ▶

The story of Inanna is similar to that of Joseph Campbell's hero. Both the hero and the heroine leave home, adventure, gain new gifts, and return. They start and end in the same place, but follow different paths. In a similar way, both the Sun and Moon Salutations begin and end in Mountain Pose, a foundational pose representing the essential self. Their journeys, however, are fundamentally different. The Sun Salutation involves stepping out to take on life's challenges, while the Moon Salutation represents descent, dropping down toward the earth and giving one's entire weight to the mystery of the unknown. Both of these paths have their place and purpose.

Any woman who undertakes the journey to wholeness is a heroine. All women who choose to raise a child, love another, care for a dying parent, be vulnerable, or speak their truth in the face of the unknown, are brave souls on this planet. Practicing the Moon Salutation helps us integrate and surrender to the mystery, to integrate life's ups and downs so common to our lives.

It is difficult to predict when we might be called to follow the path of deep surrender. Through practicing the Moon Salutation, we honor the downward and corresponding upward journeys, acknowledging the wisdom to be gained by integrating both dark and light.

25
BALANCING UPPER AND LOWER CHAKRAS

Walking in beauty does not signify
The capacity of walking on water,
But walking with your feet firmly
Planted on the ground while your
Eyes are fixed on the stars
And your heart compassionately
Breathes with the rest of creation.

~ Henryk Skolimowski, *EcoYoga: Practice and Meditations*
for Walking in Beauty on the Earth

The Moon Salutation connects us deeply into the earth while at the same time opening our consciousness to the heavens. It balances upper and lower chakras, earth and sky. The Moon Salutation strengthens the lower chakras while also allowing earth energy to move through the body and beyond. The energy that is awakened in the pelvis and belly moves up to the heart and is radiated in all directions.

Yoga teacher Satya Rita Milleli related this story of how she used the Moon Salutation to help her become more grounded in her body and thus to integrate the bliss state she was experiencing.

Once during meditation I went into pure spirit energy and
felt myself moving away from the group. I went into a bliss

*state, an experience I had never had that deeply in medita-
tion. I felt I did not want to leave that spirit realm.*

*When the meditation was over, I had to drive home,
but I was very much out of my body. I knew I had to ground
myself, so I did the Moon Salutation. It helped me to come
back into my body without taking away the sense of bliss.*

*For me, the Moon Salutation represents Shakti com-
ing into the Mother Earth. It's the earth energy that we
are receiving from the planet. It strengthens me through its
grounding. Shiva is about moving up into higher chakras;
it's the pure bliss state, but Shakti makes it present and
physical. The Moon Salutation has the whole opening in
the lower chakras, which makes it expanding, opening, and
grounding.*

*This experience corresponds with the intention of my
practice. I want to be fully present physically and fully
divine at the same time. I want to move into bliss and stay
grounded.*

As Satya points out, the Moon Salutation connects us to
the earth body as well as to our own spirit body. As the pelvis is
opened in the squats, the body is literally close to the earth; we
feel its energy rising through the legs and into the torso.

One of the co-creators of the Moon Salutation, Deva Parnell,
explained to me the way that the Moon Salutation expresses the
two poles of being as expressed in Yogic philosophy: *prakriti* and
purusha. Here is Deva as she explains:

*Spirit made manifest is the feminine while the unmanifest
is male. The earth is the mother, the physical manifestation.
The sky is the male principle, the unmanifest. These polarities come from the ancient understandings of purusha, or
spirit, and prakriti, or matter. After honoring the self in
the form of the physical body the tips of the fingers point
down to honor the earth. They then circle up to honor the
heavens, the unmanifest male.*

▼   ▼   ▼

When I was in my 20s examining the Judeo-Christian tradition in which I had been raised, I saw the many ways it denigrated the feminine and the earth. The Judeo-Christian Bible documents ancient sites of tree worship on hillsides being torn down, those who honored Goddesses being seen as worshipping false prophets, and has no feminine parallel to the male-oriented Lord's Prayer from the book of Matthew. I had spent my life reciting "Our Father which art in heaven" and I longed for a feminine equivalent. I vowed that I would not recite this prayer again until I had an equally potent prayer, "Our Mother who art in the earth."

Almost two decades later this time came, when I felt a profoundly powerful relationship with nature, when I could hear the trees and the ocean speaking to me, and when I felt a powerful connection to Divine Mother, to the voice of Shakti or Love speaking to me through nature and through my body in ways that I knew to be true. This came primarily through following the call to do my dissertation research on Green Yoga (which will have to remain the topic of a future book) but also through Yoga in general, through women's circles and women's spirituality, and the Moon Salutation. One day I knew I was so strongly connected to earth in my ongoing embodied prayer that I could now say the "Our Father" prayer as well.[101]

To me, this is becoming whole ~ filling in the missing pieces of embodiment so that it is possible to reclaim rather than reject gifts from our childhood. We need the earth and we need the sky. We need our mothers and we need our fathers. We need to be fully embodied and at the same time fully divine.

---

101. My favorite version is the Aramaic translation by Neil Douglas-Klotz, from *Prayers of the Cosmos: Meditations on the Aramaic Words of Jesus* (New York: Harper Collins, 1990), 41.

26

YIN, YANG, AND BEYOND ~ GROWING OUR GENDER MUSCLES

There is a man in the inner depths of every woman, and a woman in the inner depths of every man. This truth dawned in the meditation of the great saints and seers eons ago. This is what the Ardhanariswara (half God and half Goddess) concept in the Hindu faith signifies. Whether you are a woman or a man, your real humanity will come to light only when the feminine and masculine qualities within you are balanced.

~ Ammachi, *The Awakening of Universal Motherhood*

So many of us as children received limiting messages regarding our gender. As girls we were told not to be too pushy, not to speak up. We received subtle and not-so-subtle messages not to be smart. Our male friends were told not to cry, not to be tender. Nobody wants to be put in a box. Men don't want to have to be strong all the time. Women don't want to be limited to positions of mind-numbing inferiority. And wherever we are on the gender spectrum, we all want to be able to express our full range of qualities, dark and light, humble and proud, strong and tender. We all need the freedom to show up fully to give our gifts.

Gender stereotypes create havoc, pain, and limitations on full self-expression, especially for those among us who conform the least to the gender we were assigned at birth. Children who don't fit into expected gender norms may face severe consequences, including being teased, excluded, bullied, and much worse. As the hate-crime rate in the United States sadly shows, transgender people (and especially trans-women of color) are subject to harassment, rape, and murder at much higher rates than the general population.

Joan of Arc was a threat to the British hierarchy because her spiritual intuition so effectively aided the French on the battlefield. And yet, the crime for which she was convicted and burned was cross-dressing as a man. This is the ultimate sin to patriarchy, the supposed audacity of a woman to take on the characteristics, and through them the privilege, of a man. Lesbian, gay, bisexual, transgender, and intersex people challenge gender stereotypes, and often bear the brunt of a misogynistic culture which sees them as a profound threat.

Whether or not we are subject to physical violence as a result of our gender expression, rigid gender norms affect all of us. Limited gender expression stamps out healthy creativity, as our soul knows no such boundaries. Today, more and more people desire to express the full range of human expression, whether considered traditionally masculine or feminine.

For many, the model of *yin* and *yang* provides a useful construct within which to bring awareness to the play of opposites and polarity in our lives. Certified Yoga Therapist Lydie Lakshmi Ometto shares how she loves to play with all polarities in her Yoga practice:

Exploring opposites to bring a state of equilibrium in the body fascinates me. I play in this field in all aspects of my personal and professional life. The moon and the sun, surrender and effort, yin and yang, contraction and expansion, light and dark, female and male, fire and water, and so many more. Through those explorations I strive to recognize the full benefits of both sides of all spectrums and how they complement each other in a multitude of ways, considering the multi-dimensional beings that we are.

The Moon Salutation helps us to expand our gender muscles by opening us to a wide range of expression ‑ fierce and gentle, strong and soft, protective and quiet. John Willey, a former Director of Yoga Teacher Training at Kripalu, describes how he is committed to creating balance in his approach toward life, and how the Moon Salutation helps him to do that:

> *When I think about practicing the Moon Salutation as a man, I know that there needs to be balance in my life, and I believe that the Moon Salutation provides that balance. If I am looking for completeness, if I am looking to develop all aspects of awareness in my consciousness, then I need to think of all directions. I need to think in a sphere.*
>
> *The two series together become a very powerful sadhana (practice) for me. For a while I did the Sun Salutation followed by the Moon Salutation and that was my sadhana. For me both salutations have a warrioresque energy. In the Sun Salutation the warrior is in expression. In the Moon Salutation it is in internal receptivity.*
>
> *The Moon Salutation gives you a transformative boost. How often do we stop, stand still, and open laterally? Really, it makes you think spherically rather than linearly.*

Expression and receptivity, the right and left hemispheres of our brain, waking and sleeping modes of being, passive and active are all polarities on which to balance and draw. A healthy human flexibly moves between and through these phases of being. Limiting ourselves to only one aspect of any polarity creates an unhealthy imbalance.

I love that the Vedic tradition includes a full range of possible role models for gender expression. The Hindu Goddess encompasses dark and light, good and bad, fierce and gentle in her many aspects. Kali is dark and ferocious, fearsome and wild. Lakshmi is beautiful and peaceful, tranquil and abundant. Saraswati is meditative and creative, lyrical and thoughtful. I like to think of a rainbow spectrum of expression within, around, and between genders. We are all a rainbow of qualities, interests, skills, and abilities that overlap within and among genders. No two people are the same in their expression or experience of gender.

It's helpful to reflect on our gender expression in order to continually break out of the narrow definitions of femininity and masculinity we have inherited. Are we constantly expanding the edges of our own concept of ourselves? How do we embody strength, ferocity, power? How do we express gentleness and tenderness? Where are we wild, loving, and playful? How are we steady, reliable, trustworthy? Do our communities include those who are not in the middle of the norm of the gender spectrum, and do we embrace their gifts?

We all work with our own rainbow spectrum of gender. We all need to explore and expand to create balance. We need to practice getting out of the box and thinking more broadly, moving beyond the social constructs we have been given. The Moon Salutation combined with supportive, inquiring community can help us to do that.

27

MEN AND MOON SALUTATIONS

The Moon Salutation is my husband's favorite flow. Every time he comes to my Yoga class he asks me to teach it.

~ Susan Kirinich, Kripalu Yoga Teacher

Men at this time in history are also healing their relationship to feminine aspects of being and to the Goddess. As the Moon Salutation was created by and for women, more attention has been given so far to women's than to men's experience of it. Yet it is also powerful for men.

Carl Jung addressed the role of women's mysteries in men's development in his discussion of the ancient Greek Demeter/ Kore (Persephone) rituals. Demeter was the Goddess of agriculture and fertility who descended to the underworld to recover her lost daughter Persephone, who had been abducted. Jung said that while these festivals of dancing during the fall planting were "too feminine" to have been created by men, they had lasting and abiding significance for men through their ability to enrich and widen the psyche.[102] Similarly, participating in the female mystery of the Moon Salutation enriches and widens the psyche of modern-day men.

In teaching the Moon Salutation in mixed groups of women and men, teachers are careful to use inclusive language. For

---

102. Carl Gustav Jung, *Aspects of the Feminine* (Princeton, NJ: Princeton University Press, 1982).

example, I recommend using the word "center" instead of "womb space," and "pelvic floor" instead of *yoni*."

Yoga retreat leader Tracie Sage describes the different responses men and women may have to this flow, and how she nuances her language to match the students:

> *My female students always love the Moon Salutation immediately and my men students don't always love it right away. It really depends. When I teach it to men I don't emphasize female empowerment. I bring out the creative aspects of the sequence, and the feminine aspects of our being,*
>
> *I'm careful not to use language that would make men feel left out, excluded in a subtle way, as if there were something wrong with being masculine.*

I have been very touched by the men in my classes who have learned the Moon Salutation, and by the men with whom I have spoken about what it means to them. Kripalu Yoga Teacher Dave Seaman shared with me how he uses the Moon Salutation in his own practice to honor feminine power. "I like to do the flow myself whenever there is a full moon. I might go out and do it in the backyard. For me it's a way of honoring the female cycle, the power of birth and fertility." While Dave himself may not experience personally the mystery of the female cycle, he chooses to honor its power in this way.

With his students Dave emphasizes the masculine and feminine in all of us. "When I teach it I explain to my students that it is about the female energy in all of us, that we all have both a feminine and a masculine side." Both men and women at this time are striving to reintegrate and strengthen all aspects of our being.

Yoga teacher David Lurey guides the Moon Salutation on new and full moons, as well as using it in his own personal practice when drawn.

> *The Moon Salutation has become an essential part of my teaching whenever it fits the moon cycle. I used it recently in my men's circle as an embodiment practice to bring the group into a feeling state.*

It was hard to watch how many of the men struggled with the flow of it and with the range of motion in the hips. It was clear that repetition of the Moon Salute would do them well. We made three full cycles that night and all the men commented they felt 'dropped into the lunar ways' :-)

I especially love to guide Moon Salutes outside under the full moon during our teacher trainings and on retreats. It's always magical, allowing us to physically and energetically connect to the moon.

However, in full transparency, I always feel like I lead the sequence a bit "masculine" or linear. I'm always searching to bring the right tone, voice and speed to make the sequence juicy and lunar, but that's not easy for me.

Here David makes a point worth noting. While a man may devotedly practice the Moon Salutation, it may look and feel differently on his body than on a woman's body. I know David well and know him to be a juicy and lunar person, a soulful guitarist and *bhakti* singer, as well as a devoted husband and father.

But perhaps the Moon Salutation *does* look more linear and more masculine on his body, and maybe that's okay. I've noticed this in others, being amazed at how masculine the flow can sometimes look. I remember watching a leading male Yoga teacher in Full Squat Pose and thinking he looked like a Samurai warrior ~ definitely not the feminine Goddess I feel myself to be in that pose. To me this is natural and fine. Men still reap the physical benefits of opening laterally and dropping into the hips, and the spiritual benefits of connecting with the moon, no matter how linear or masculine the flow may feel for them.

As women today empower ourselves and work to create peace in the world, men who are committed to a similar healing path often become powerful allies. Megha Nancy Buttenheim, one of the co-creators of the Moon Salutation, describes how men participated in the original Women and Yoga series as a way of creating solidarity and showing their support:

One of the most beautiful parts along with the Moon Salute itself was that we invited the brothers to come in in silence. They were all dressed in white and would sing this beautiful chant. "Oh my Mother, I love you," and then we would chant back and forth. Everybody was crying and praying and thanking one another for our shared humanity.

Men who practice Moon Salutations model to other men that women matter, that lunar values matter. As women, we cannot change society alone. We need our gentle male friends to stand with us in embracing the fullness of the moon and her ways. Men practicing Moon Salutations leads to peace ~ peace within men, and peace between men and women.

28

PEACE PRAYERS ~ TWO NEW VARIATIONS

Blessed is the light, blessed is the darkness,
but blessed above all else is peace.

~ Marge Piercy, *The Art of Blessing the Day:*
Poems with a Jewish Theme

No Yoga flow is a static entity that remains the same forever. A sequence of poses is a living entity, breathing and moving among those who practice it. As people with different needs take on a Yoga flow, they naturally evolve the movements, changing them to fit their bodies, their life experiences, and the needs of their communities. New flows can come from deep intuition, from a response to a challenge or dilemma, or simply from observing the changing needs of a population of practitioners.

As I was completing this book two new flows were given to me, both of which evoked a deep sense of peace. One came as a direct transmission during meditation at the epicenter of my menopause transition, unexpected and unrequested. After meditation I wrote the sequence in my journal, then got up and did the movements. I loved the feeling of the flow on my body, the profound sense of connection to the sacred space around me. I was grateful for that gift, as I was barely sleeping that month, and needed something to hang onto for my sanity.

The other flow came in response to a request for stories from practitioners and teachers of the Moon Salutation. Yoga Teacher and Nonprofit Consultant Debra McKnight Higgins shared how she created a special version of the Moon Salutation in response to the events of 9/11 and the increasing militarism of our country. Her story demonstrates a genuine response to a collective trauma and the desire to create a more peaceful outcome. This is the ultimate intention of the Moon Salutation ~ to generate wholeness, balance, and peace in those who practice it, and from there to spread these qualities in the world more widely.

MOTHER MARY MOON SALUTATION

I believe that this sequence was sent as a gift from Mother Mary to all women. I highly recommend the Mother Mary Moon Salutation for menopause, but it can be practiced at any time of life. The movements invite a full delicious breath and direct our gaze to connect with the beauty of the universe around us. I invite you to practice it with me on our website, www.MoonSalutations.com. This flow feels natural and soft on the body, but is complex in its written form. Such is the way of movement! I highly recommend that you view the video on the website in order to get a feel for it.

However, for those who wish written directions, here are guideposts:

Mother Mary Moon Salutation Flow:

1. Begin in Mountain Pose. Allow yourself to feel grounded and open. Inhale arms up overhead to Temple.

2. Flow into Crescent Moon left as you exhale, then inhale back up, exhale hands to belly, then inhale back up.

3. Repeat Crescent Moon to the right, inhale up, exhale hands to belly, and inhale up.

4. Exhale, begin Goddess Flow.

   a. Step the left leg to the side, bending both knees, and gently let the arms flow down over the crown chakra and mid-body as if tracing the shape of the energy field, then let them flow down and out toward the earth, just in front of the thighs. Look ahead as you exhale.

b. Inhale, straighten the knees, and sweep the arms up over head with the breath. Open the eyes fully and look slightly up on the inhale.

c. Arm variation: On the exhale, hands can touch each other in prayer position and move straight down through the center of the body, sweeping out toward the earth when you reach the pelvis.

d. Continue Goddess Flow with breath and arms three times. Receive healing and blessing for your body.

e. Complete Goddess Flow on an exhale.

5. Inhale, prepare for Triangle Flow.

a. Left foot turns out, right foot turns in, both arms sweep overhead.

b. Exhale, left arm sweeps left then down toward the ground just in front of the left shin, torso follows to the left for triangle pose, hips remain open forward. Right arm remains pointing toward the sky, then complete the exhalation as you sweep the right arm 90 degrees so that it comes parallel to the ground. Look up slightly under your right arm if that works for your neck, otherwise look forward. If any pain, look down.

c. Inhale, come back up to standing by lifting the torso while rotating the arms. Right arm circles down towards the earth to end up just in front of the hips, left arm bends at the elbow and lifts up toward the sky. Eyes follow the left hand up at the completion of the exhalation.

d. Continue this Triangle Flow three times. Feel the freedom of your body as it moves.

e. Complete Triangle Flow on an exhale with left arm down.

6. Shorten the stance slightly for Pyramid Pose. Rotate the hips to face left, as square as is possible. Hands may remain touching the earth, or arms come behind the back, either in reverse prayer (palms touching, fingers pointing towards the shoulders) or holding wrists. Take three slow breaths in and out. Allow mind and heart to become quiet.

7. Inhale, prepare for Extended Side Angle Flow.

   a. Place hands on the ground on either side of your front (left) leg, step your right leg a little farther back, keeping both heels on the ground. Drop your hips a little bit, deepening the lunge.

   b. Then exhale, circling the right arm first down toward the ground and then across the upper body and reaching left into Side Angle Pose.

   c. Inhale, draw the right shoulder back, the gaze up and heart forward, and continue the circle of the right arm up and back toward your back leg. Let your gaze follow the arm all of the way around up towards the sky, then to the right, and then down again towards the earth.

   d. Continue with three Extended Side Angle Flows. Allow yourself to take in the universe that surrounds you.

   e. End with an exhale, coming into a lunge facing left, one hand on either side of the front knee, head drops down.

8. Inhale, turn the body to face forward, coming into Side Lunge. Exhale, hands to the ground. Allow yourself to feel that the earth is your companion. Continue for three complete rounds of breath, in and out. Option: If this pose is not kind to your knees or hips, feel free to omit and go directly into Full Squat from the previous pose.

9. Full Squat Pose, three full breaths in and out. Rest deeply.

10. Inhale, Side Lunge on the other side. Right leg is bent, left leg extends.

11. Inhale, prepare for Extended Side Angle Flow on the second side. Turn to the right and scoop the arm down, forward and around in a circle, three times.

12. Inhale, prepare for Pyramid Pose on the second side, arms in your chosen position. Three long slow breaths.

13. Inhale, prepare for Triangle Flow on the second side by lifting the torso, left arm stays down and comes slightly behind the hips, right arm bends at the elbow and comes gently up overhead, eyes up at the hand. Then flow in and out of triangle as above, three breaths, ending on an exhale.

14. Inhale prepare for Goddess Flow by turning both feet to face forward and bringing both arms overhead. Continue through three rounds of Goddess Flow moving through your chosen hand positions.

15. Crescent Moon Pose Flow at the end is different than the beginning of this flow. First inhale into Temple with both arms overhead and feet stepping together. Then exhale right arm stays overhead and bends left, left arm sweeps down and hand comes just in front of the body. Inhale both arms overhead. Exhale repeat to the other side. Inhale back up.

16. Exhale, complete Mother Mary Moon Salutation.

This may also be adapted to your favorite other Moon Salutation. The possibilities are infinite.

MOON SALUTATION AS A PEACE PRAYER

The moon and the Moon Salutation call us to a state of peace ~ both within ourselves and also as a prayerful intention for peace among all beings. Yoga Teacher and Nonprofit Consultant Debra McKnight Higgins shares how she used the Moon Salutation as a peace prayer during a time of increasing hostility among nations:

After the tragedy of 9/11 and the onset of our country's violence and expansion of war toward others, I was called to become a more active peacemaker for all beings and for the earth. I now use my practice as a way to ground and dispel feelings of fear and anger and to express prayers of peace and love.

During the same time period a dear friend from my meditation group died of breast cancer. A songwriter and beautiful artist, Heather Childs shared her music with us during daylong retreats and gatherings. Her last album and signature song is called "Peace Prayer." Since she could never be a mother, her songs were her children.

My connection with spirit led me to simplify and choreograph the Moon Salutation to Heather's music. During those turbulent times after 9/11 and again recently, I shared the Moon Salutation in this way with women on retreat in the woods, with my Yoga students, and many others along the path. The prayer often brings tears of happiness, as an expression of hope and possibility.

Here are the words to this poem taken loosely from the *Rig Veda*:

May peace be in the universe.
May peace fill all the skies.
May peace be in the winds.
May peace be over all the earth.

May the animals and plants have peace.
May the holy ones have peace.
May they bless us with peace.
May they bless us with peace.

~ Heather Childs,[103]

---

103. Heather Childs. *Peace Prayer.* (Rochester, Michigan, Heather Childs, 1998), compact disc.

29

LIVING AS A DAUGHTER
OF THE MOON

When I told a friend I was writing this book, she exclaimed, "Why, you're a daughter of the moon!" "What does that mean?" I asked her.

"I have no idea," she replied, "I just know that that's what you are."

And so I began to ponder what it meant. What does it mean to claim the moon as guide and protector, to live in its soft light, to go at its pace? What does it mean to embrace the dark as well as the light? What does it mean for our movements to be a prayer for peace?

The moon teaches me not to rush. This has been a hard lesson. As someone who was taught to achieve and to measure my worthiness in rule-following and outward accomplishments, it has taken many decades to relax into a slower pace, the pace of my heart, my soul, and the moon.

The moon reminds me ~ whatever my current life moment ~ that everything is temporary. This day will be gone soon, so I choose to receive its gifts to the fullest. It has taken me several decades to truly receive the lessons the Moon Salutation and this book have for me. But I am learning, slowly. I learn not to force life. I can't make things happen when they're not ready. Nature will not be rushed.

In some ways, I have always been a daughter of the moon. I have always loved nature, poetry, and dance. I love water, swimming, and the ocean ~ lunar symbols for many. My dream of women dancing over the field with radiant flowers and radiant earth spoke of the earthy, radiant essence of my soul. But the lessons of receiving, resting, and relaxing into soulfulness have been hard-earned for me.

I continue to rely on the physical presence and light of the moon to soften and gentle me. Whenever I see the moon I look up to receive her surprising beauty. The moon changes at a pace we don't always expect, and if I'm not totally tracking her phases, she can catch me off guard. I see her after new moon, low and delicate on the horizon, following the setting sun. Or I see her as she approaches full moon, larger and gathering power.

If I wake in the middle of the night on full moon I meditate outside, bathing in her light and sitting with the plants – who seem to relish the moonlight as much as I do. I love these unexpected visits. Sometimes I plan a hike or walk to a place where I know I can sit and meditate with the rising full moon, or with the new moon as she sets. More often I am surprised and grateful.

Sometimes I plan retreats around the moon, wanting my participants to share in the ecstasy of her fullness with dance or chanting. I have also led retreats on the new moon, naming and integrating the vortex of emptiness and dark potential through which we are passing together.

From my journal in 1998:

Walking home from Yoga class, I see a crescent-shaped, reddish sliver of moon. I am at first taken aback by its strange color and placement. I pause to take in the sight. My years of studying math and physics leap to mind, and I find myself geometrically calculating how the moon could be at that height in the sky, where it must be in its monthly cycle, its angular relation to the sun.

As my analytically curious mind presses to understand, another part of my mind is captured by its mystery – the surprise of the moon's eerie and beautiful appearance this night. The poet, the muse, does not seek to dismiss through knowing but prefers to rest in beauty, to appreciate, to be moved and inspired.

I reflect on the consequences of our several-millennia-long love affair with the sun at the near exclusion of the moon. We worship the constancy, orderliness, and accomplishments of the sun gods at the expense of the mystery, subtlety, and playfulness of the moon goddesses. What might our world be like if we honored the powers of both moon and sun?

Twenty years later I am more familiar with the moon. I have softened into her ways. The moon is just there, received as a beauty or a presence. I have grown over the past 20 years. I have married, divorced, and married again. I have gone through menopause. I have wanted to have a baby, and finally decided not to. I've experienced the death of my mom, and am just beginning to integrate the meaning of her life for me. I have surrendered to many difficult experiences, and worked with the Goddess to improve or radically change others. I have received incredible gifts, incredible blessings.

Other women, too, speak of how the moon has touched their souls and melted hard places within that kept them separate from their true essence. Yoga Teacher Malú Doherty recounts how the moon touched her heart, transforming it forever:

The first time I felt the awe and magnificence of the moon was eight years ago when I was driving home after a month at the beach. It was early morning, dark, and hard to leave that month of warm sun. As I turned onto the six-mile drive I was struck by the full moon, hovering large, just above the ocean and waiting to set.

The moon cast a path of light across the water. Like a laser beam it went straight into my heart. In an instant, I fell into awe. Iciness melted inside me. It was a beginning, a start of some journey I didn't yet understand. I couldn't keep the tears from coming. I told myself it had to do with returning from my trip, but I knew it was so much more. Something was calling me to my heart, to embrace myself in my aging body and graying hair. It felt like a call to love the woman and the healer I was becoming.

The soft light carried a message, not in words but in feeling. 'I am the embodiment of a woman's energy, love, sensuality and wisdom. Hold yourself gently. Don't turn away. Embrace what's here and let it be seen.' It was only a few minutes, but something changed in me forever. I felt softness, reverence, and a connection with universal love that has never left me.

Today, I teach Yoga and offer energy healing using moonstone, envisioning the light in me and in others. I still see it like I did that morning, a moonbeam traveling across the ocean, blessing everything above and below it, heading straight for the heart. I believe that same light brings heal-ing to everyone's heart.

The light of the moon reaches across time and space to touch not only human hearts but to speak to the waters, the plants, and the animals. Dolphins dance with her, flowers open to her. Says Yoga Instructor Kendra West:

My passion for the moon resides with the brightest light in my heart. It represents my sensual sweetness and fills my soul with the quiet of night and with the grace of movement that flows and heals me at my deep emotional core.

Becoming a daughter of the moon means listening to intu-ition, to the voice of the soul. It means slowing down enough so that the soul can actually be heard. The soul moves at a slower pace than the mind. Becoming a daughter of the moon means following the pace of the soul. Becoming a daughter of the moon means sitting in circles on new or full moons, joining with others to celebrate the lunar ways. It means honoring our bodies, our lives, our needs. It means telling our stories and sharing them with others, including the painful parts. It means helping each other as women to heal, whatever that takes.

Becoming a daughter of the moon means also becoming a daughter of the earth. We connect with our true mother, this earth, which holds and grounds all our experiences. We learn to love the hills, plants, and flowers. We talk to the trees, commune with the stars. We become friends with earth and sky, heaven and earth.

Living as a daughter of the moon is an ongoing journey. It is that soulful place of earth connection. It is making love to life itself, or to a specific beloved. It is meditating with no goal other than presence, openness. It is being out in nature, doing nothing, placing one's back on the earth, heart to the sky. It is dancing at night, flowing in a circle, listening to inspiration.

What does the moon want to say? "You are my beloved. You are Divine Love. You are held. You are beautiful, whole, and pure. You are earth. You are always with me in my heart. Don't forget your true home and your true mother. Be at peace."

Blessed Be!

NEXT STEPS

1. If you enjoyed this book, please consider leaving a review on your favorite book review site or store.

2. It would be a great favor to me if you would pass this book on or purchase an additional copy for your Yoga teacher or Yoga practitioner friend.

2. For videos, more feminine-honoring practices, and support in bringing this into the world, visit www.MoonSalutations.com

CONTRIBUTORS

Thank you to all of the women and men who contributed to this book. You gave generously of your time, energy, and love so that I could share your stories and teaching with others. Thank you for the many interviews and conversations we had and for the emails, stories, and poems you sent. The wisdom you shared greatly expanded the breadth of this work.

MOON SALUTATION CO-CREATORS

Megha Nancy Buttenheim, www.letyouryogadance.com
Acharya Deva Parnell, www.disoveryyoga.com
Harriet L. Russell (Bhumi), www.bhumiyoga.com
Patricia "Niti" Seip Martin, www.doingwellyoga.com

BOOK CONTRIBUTORS

Barbara Badger
Libby Cox, www.twobirdsyogatraining.com
Jenny Berthiaume
Mary Lou Buck, www.cornwellcenter.org/staff
Martha Chabinsky
Carol P. Christ, www.goddessariadne.org
Carly Conatser, Instagram: carlyyogipoet
Malú Doherty, www.maludoherty.com
Erin Dowd, www.adaptiveyogaforall.com
Mary Lynn Fitton, www.theartofyogaproject.org
Deborah Foss, www.reclaimyourlight.net
Beth Good Wadden, www.heartsongyoga.com
Deah Jenkins, www.1lightwellness

Chris Keyser
Sue Kirinich, www.sueyoga.com
Valerie Kit Love, www.metromystic@gmail.com
Stacey Louise, www.inspiredkidsyoga.com.au
Sudha Carolyn Lundeen, www.sudhalundeen.com
David Lurey, www.findbalance.net
Chaitra Makam, www.heartfulnessinstitute.org
Debra McKnight Higgins, www.mcknighthiggins.com
Satya Rita Milleli
Richard Miller, www.irest.org
Mirella Nicholson
Lydie Lakshmi Ometto, www.lydieometto.com
Arisika Razak, www.eastbaymeditation.org
Valerie Renwick
Dave Seaman
Tracie Sage, www.traciesage.com
Elizabeth Shillington
Kendra West, www.earthelementsyoga.com
John Willey
Esther Wyss-Flamm, www.estherwyssflamm.com

PHOTO MODELS

Denise Alston, www.spirit1styoga.com
Maria Arvayo, www.studioyoga.space
Laura Hernandez, www.yogaetmouvement.com
Reed Kolber, www.honeycombhealing.com
Stacey Louise, www.inspiredkidsyoga.com.au
Anh Chi Pham, www.chiyogawellness.com

ACKNOWLEDGMENTS

I would first like to thank all of my teachers, the many women and men who have guided me along the way, who have been companions on the soul journey of awakening. Thank you to the many who guided me personally in meditation, Yoga, and simply being an awakening spirit in a human body. My teachers are also all of those who have sat with me in sacred circle, been in Quaker Worship with me, meditated with me, or practiced Yoga with me, as well as my students, friends, colleagues, and all those who shared with me in preparation for this book.

In particular, I want to thank all of the teachers, founders, board members, and innumerable volunteers over many decades at the Kripalu Center for Yoga and Health. The teachings you nurtured and continue to live and spread in the world have provided fertile ground for my understanding and growth as a yogini. I would not be who I am without you.

Specifically, I give appreciation to Melanie Armstrong-King and Ann Greene, who were my first Yoga teacher trainers at Kripalu. Tarika Diane Damelio wisely directed the Women and Yoga Program I attended. Rudy Pierce gave exceptional training in Yoga teacher mentoring, which still forms the basis of much of my work.

To Jalaja Bonheim, thank you for inspirational teaching of the Divine Mother and for naming my readiness for this journey many, many years ago. To Shannon Peck, thank you for your light-filled teaching on the power of love and for nurturing my spirit. To Elaine Emily, thank you for being a faithful friend and spiritual elder over many decades, always holding space for what is wanting to emerge. To Blake Arnall, thank you for being a tender companion in this process through our spirit circle with

Elaine. I send deep appreciation and gratitude also to Rachael Jayne Groover for your friendship, your mentoring, and for being such a powerful model of feminine embodiment.

The California Institute of Integral Studies provided a perfect breeding ground for the early stages of this research through its support of embodied and deeply transformative scholarship. Many professors encouraged my creativity and vision while showing me how to be an ethically-grounded and intelligent researcher. Thank you to Connie Jones, Jim Ryan, Carol Whitfield, Jorge Ferrer, Mara Keller, Eahr Joan, and Carolyn Foster. I was blessed that CIIS faculty member Stuart Sovatsky was also a disciple of Swami Kripalu. Stuart gave insightful perspectives on an early version of this work. Thank you also to Carol Christ, whose course "Rebirth of the Goddess" was the first incubator for the insights and the poem that later grew into this book.

I give special thanks to the Northern California Kripalu Yoga Teachers Group of the 1990s. They offered companionship on the path and supported the early stages of this project. Particular thanks go to Sita Packer and Path Star who dialogued with me at critical junctures.

A deep bow of appreciation to Lydie Lakshmi Ometto, whose "Swimming with the Dolphins and Yoga Retreat" two years ago in the Bahamas provided the perfect space for me to get clear which book to complete first. I never wavered after receiving that guidance.

A big debt of gratitude to Tom Bird, my writing coach, who helped me finally birth the new material and new structure for this book that had been wanting to emerge for so long. Thank you for holding space for me to relax and write. My soul is forever grateful.

Thank you to Jessica Hadari and to the entire community of FemTalks for providing a container for my writing over the past year through retreat days and sisterminds. It meant more than I can say to have a place to read what was being birthed and to feel it received in your hearts.

Thank you to Chris Chapple for saying that 20 years to birth a solo book is about right. You are a shining light and a role model to me, always a source of encouragement. Your words help me to smile and take a deep breath.

To Ivy Ingram, thank you for your inspired editing. It is always a pleasure and a joy working with you. To Erin Dowd, thank you for your detailed comments and your commitment to making Yoga so accessible. To Wendy Wiltrout, thank you for meticulous administrative and editorial support. I couldn't do this work without you.

Thank you to Beth Barany for your helpful suggestions about the book organization and Table of Contents. Thank you to Charles Clendenin, Sharon Delap, Abe Doherty, Simon Graveline, Jim Otis, Maggie Weber-Striplin, and Meghan Westlander for their generous time in taking the photos that became the drawings in this book. Thank you to a sweet team of artists and graphic designers Priyanka Bose, Rumi Das, Sharon Delap, Janani Chathubhashini Narahenpita, and Sasmita Adi Nugraha. Sharon is also the one who showed me the Moon Salutation and went with me on my first Yoga journey 25 years ago. Thank you!

I give deep gratitude to my co-housing community, whose support networks and friendly dinners allowed me to share that I was "almost done" more times than any of us care to remember. You were loving with me throughout, reminding me that I could be the same for myself.

Thank you to my mom (now an ancestor) for being open to healing with me. Thank you to my dad for gracefully allowing me to share our story, even when it isn't comfortable. Thank you to my sister Diane for always supporting my work and teaching. Thank you to "Ginni" (Virginia) Neil for coming into our lives at the perfect moment.

Thank you to my sisters and brothers at the Heartfulness Institute. I feel in you the heart that reaches beyond culture to speak the language of the soul. You have all my love. Thank you to Shobha Prabala for reading a good portion of the book aloud with me and discussing suggested changes.

A deep bow of gratitude to my husband, Jim Otis, who has steadfastly believed in my vision and who supported my sabbatical and spiritual retirement so that I would have the time and space to write. I treasure the creativity, freedom, and growth you nurture in me. You are a true lover of the Divine Feminine.

BIBLIOGRAPHY

Anderson, Sherry Ruth and Hopkins, Patricia. *The Feminine Face of God: The Unfolding of the Sacred in Women.* New York: Bantam Books, 1991.

Apffel-Marglin, Frederique. *The Wives of the God-King: The Rituals of the Devadasis of Puri.* New York: Oxford University Press, 1985.

Barnard, Mary. *Sappho: A Translation.* Shabhala, Boston: Shambhala Pocket Classics, 1994. Original publication 1958.

Bonheim, Jalaja. *Aphrodite's Daughters: Women's Sexual Stories and the Journey of the Soul.* New York: Fireside Books, 1997.

Buttenheim, Nancy Megha (Speaker). *Beyond Limits: Moon Series.* Lenox, MA: Kripalu Center, 1991, audiotape.

Campbell, Joseph. *The Hero with a Thousand Faces.* 2nd ed. Princeton, NJ: Princeton University Press, 1968. (Original work published 1949)

Chaudhuri, Haridas. *Being, Evolution, and Immortality: An Outline of Integral Philosophy.* Wheaton, IL: Quest Books, 1974. (Original work published 1967 under the title *The Philosophy of Integralism*)

Chen, Lijun, Jingjing Qu, and Charlie Xiang. "The Multi-functional Roles of Menstrual Blood-derived Stem Cells in Regenerative Medicine." *Stem Cell Research and Therapy* 10 (2019). https://www.ncbi.nlm.nih.gov/pmc/articles/PMC6318883/ (accessed May 13, 2019)

Chia, Mantak, and Arava, Douglas Abrams. *The Multi-Orgasmic Man.* San Francisco: HarperCollins Publishers, 1996.

Childs, Heather. *Peace Prayer.* Rochester, Michigan, Heather Childs, 1998, compact disc.

Christ, Carol P. *Rebirth of the Goddess: Finding Meaning in Feminine Spirituality.* New York: Routledge, 1997.

Christ, Carol P. *She Who Changes: Re-Imagining the Divine in the World.* New York: Palgrave Macmillan. 2003.

Cornell, Laura. "Adult Psychological Development in the Practice of Kripalu Yoga: A Jungian Perspective." *International Journal of Yoga Therapy* 8 (1998). 31-39.

Cornell, Laura. "Me Too: How I Healed from Incest to Recover the Divine Feminine Within." In *The Game Changer (Volume 3): Inspirational Stories that Changed Lives,* edited by Iman Aghay, Vancouver, Canada: Success Road Enterprises, 2018, 233-244.

Cornell, Laura, *The Moon Salutation: Expression of the Feminine in Body, Psyche, Spirit.* Emeryville, CA: Yogeshwari Arts. 2000.

Cushman, Anne. "New Light on Yoga." *Yoga Journal,* 147 (July/August, 1999). 44-49.

Desai, Yogi Amrit. *Kripalu Yoga: Meditation in Motion Book 1.* Rev. ed. Lenox, MA: Kripalu Yoga Fellowship, 1990.

Desikachar, T. K. V. *The Heart of Yoga: Developing a Personal Practice.* Rochester, VT: Inner Traditions International, 1995.

Domar, Alice D., and Kelly, Alice Lesch. *Conquering Infertility: Dr. Alice Domar's Mind/Body Guide to Enhancing Fertility and Coping with Infertility.* New York: Penguin Books, 2004.

Douglas-Klotz, Neil. *Prayers of the Cosmos: Meditations on the Aramaic Words of Jesus.* New York: Harper Collins. 1990.

Eisler, Riane. *The Chalice and the Blade: Our History, our Future.* New York: Harper Collins, 1987.

Faulds, Danna. *Into the Heart of Yoga: One Woman's Journey: A Memoir.* Greenville, Virginia: Peaceable Kingdom Books, 2011.

Feuerstein, Georg. *The Yoga Tradition: Its History, Literature, Philosophy, and Practice.* Prescott, AZ: Hohm Press, 1998.

Feuerstein, Georg. "The Origins of the Sun Salutation." *Yoga World: International Newsletter for Yoga Teachers and Students,* 8 (January-March, 1999). 8.

Friend, John. "Anjaneyasana." *Yoga Journal, 142* (September/October, 1998). 22-24.

Gadon, Elinor. "Sanctifying the Home: The Ritual Art of the Women of Bengal." In *The Sacred Dimension of Women's Experience,* edited by Elizabeth Dodson Gray, 112–118. Wellesley, MA: Roundtable Press, 1989.

Gadon, Elinor. "The Hindu Goddess Shashti: Protector of Women and Children." In *From the Realm of the Ancestors: An Anthology in Honor of Marija Gimbutas,* edited by Joan Marler, 293–308. Manchester, CT: Knowledge, Ideas and Trends, 1997.

Galland, China. *The Longing for Darkness: Tara and the Dark Madonna.* New York: Penguin Books, 1990.

Grahn, Judy. *Blood, Bread, and Roses: How Menstruation Created the World.* Boston: Beacon Press, 1993.

Jayakar, Pupul. *The Earth Mother: Legends, Ritual Arts, and Goddesses of India.* New York: Harper and Row, 1990.

Jnaneshvar, Shri. *Jnaneshwari.* Translated by V. Pradhan. Albany: State University of New York Press, 1987.

Jung, Carl Gustav. *Aspects of the Feminine.* Princeton: Princeton University Press, 1982. (Original works published 1921, 1927, 1928, 1938, and 1941)

Kamlesh D. Patel et al. *The Heartfulness Way: Heart-Based Meditations for Spiritual Transformation.* Oakland, California: New Harbinger Publications, 2018.

Kilmurray, Arthur. "Yoga for Hips and Thighs." Yoga Journal, 90 (May/June, 1989). 60- 64.

Kinsley, David. *Hindu Goddesses: Visions of the Divine Feminine in the Hindu Religious Tradition.* Berkeley: University of California Press, 1986.

Kripalu. *Yoga Teacher Training Manual.* Lenox, MA: Kripalu Center, 1995.

Iyengar, Geeta. *Yoga: A Gem for Women.* Spokane, WA: Timeless Books, 1990.

Lasater, Judith. *Relax and Renew: Restful Yoga for Stressful Times.* Berkeley, CA: Rodmell Press, 1995.

Leslie, Julia, ed. *Roles and Rituals for Hindu Women.* Cranbury, NJ: Associated University Presses, 1991.

Miller, Richard. "The Psychophysiology of Respiration: Eastern and Western Perspectives." *The Journal of the International Association of Yoga Therapists, 2* (1991). 8-23.

Miller, Richard. "Pranayama and Mudras." In Joseph LePage, *Integrative Yoga Therapy Manual.* Soquel, CA: Integrative Yoga Therapy Training Program, 1993.

Mindell, Arnold. *Dreambody: The Body's Role in Revealing the Self.* Boston: Sigo Press, 1982.

Mohan, A.G. *Yoga-Yajnavalkya.* Trans. Madras, India: Ganesh and Co, 2000.

Mookerjee, Ajit. *Kali: The Feminine Force.* Rochester, NY: Destiny Books, 1988.

Mookerjee, Ajit, & Khanna, Madhu. *The Tantric Way: Art, Science, Ritual.* London: Thames and Hudson, 1977.

Morell, Virginia. "Dolphins Could Unveil the Origins of Menopause." *Science.* July 17, 2018. https://www.sciencemag.org/news/2018/07/dolphins-could-unveil-origins-menopause (accessed January 5, 2019)

Mroz, Jacqueline. *Girl Talk: What Science Can Tell Us About Female Friendship.* New York: Seal Press, 2018.

Noble, Vicki. "The Double Goddess." Lecture given at the California Institute of Integral Studies, San Francisco, CA, March 10, 2000.

Northrup, Christiane. *Women's Bodies, Women's Wisdom: Creating Physical and Emotional Health and Healing.* Rev. ed. New York: Bantam Books, 1998.

Oxman, Thomas, M.D. "Reflections on Aging and Wisdom." *The American Journal of Geriatric Psychiatry* 26, no. 11 (November, 2018). 1108-1118.

Pant, Apa. *Surya Namaskars: An Ancient Indian Exercise.* 3rd ed. Bombay: Orient Longman, 1989. Originally published 1970.

Piercy, Marge. *The Art of Blessing the Day: Poems with a Jewish Theme.* New York: Alfred A. Knopf, 1999.

Questions on T. Krishnamacharya, answered by T. K. V. Desikachar *KYM Darshanam*, November, 1993.

Radha, Swami Shivananda. *Hatha Yoga: The Hidden Language: Symbols, Secrets, and Metaphor.* Spokane, WA: Timeless Books, 1995. (Original work published 1987)

Radhakrishnan, S. *The Bhagavadgita: With an Introductory Essay, Sanskrit Text, English Translation and Notes.* New Delhi: HarperCollins Publisher India, 1993. (Original work published 1948)

Rettner, Rachael. "Why Older Adults Are Happier." Live Science. May 29, 2013. https://www.livescience.com/34825-older-adults-happiness-negative-emotions (accessed May 13, 2019).

Roderick, Libby. "How Could Anyone Ever Tell You." If You See a Dream. Anchorage, Alaska: Turtle Island Records (1990), compact disc.

Sarasohn, Lisa. "Honoring the Belly." *Yoga Journal, 121* (July/August, 1993). 76-85.

Saraswati, Swami Satyananda. *Asana, Pranayama, Mudra, Bandha.* Bihar, India: Yoga Publications Trust, 1963.

Saraswati, Swami Satyananda. *Surya Namaskara: A Technique of Solar Visualization.* Bihar, India: Bihar School of Yoga, 1973.

Satprakashananda, Swami. *The Goal and the Way.* St. Louis, MO: The Vedanta Society of St. Louis, 1977.

Singleton, Mark. *Yoga Body: The Origins of Modern Posture Practice.* New York: Oxford University Press, 2010.

Sjoman, N. E. *The Yoga Tradition of the Mysore Palace.* New Delhi, India: Shakti Malik Abhinav Publications, 1996.

Sovatsky, Stuart. *Eros, Consciousness, and Kundalini: Deepening Sensuality Through Tantric Celibacy and Spiritual Intimacy.* Rochester, VT: Park Street Press, 1994.

Sovatsky, Stuart. *Words from the Soul: Time, East/West Spirituality, and Psychotherapeutic Narrative.* New York: State University of New York Press, 1998.

Sparrowe, Linda. *The Woman's Book of Yoga and Health: A Lifelong Guide to Wellness: With Yoga Sequences by Patricia Walden.* Boston: Shambhala, 2002.

Sri Mata Amritanandamayi Devi (also known as Amma). *The Awakening of Universal Motherhood: Geneva Speech.* 2nd ed. Kerala, India: Mata Amritanandamayi Mission Trust, 2004.

Svatmarama, Shri. *Hathapradipika.* Translated by Gharote, Manmath, and Devnath, Parimal. Lonavla, India: Lonavla Yoga Institute, 2001.

Taylor, Shelley E. et al. "Biobehavioral Responses to Stress in Females: Tend-and-Befriend, Not Fight-or-Flight." *Psychological Review* 107, No. 3 (2000). 411-429.

Taylor, Shelley E. *The Tending Instinct: How Nurturing is Essential for Who We Are and How We Live.* Kindle Edition. New York: USA MacMillan, 2002.

Wolkstein, Diane & Kramer, Samuel Noah. *Inanna: Queen of Heaven and Earth: Her Stories and Hymns from Sumer.* New York: Harper and Row, 1983.

Woodman, Marion. *The Owl was a Baker's Daughter: Obesity, Anorexia Nervosa and the Repressed Feminine.* Toronto: Inner City Books, 1980.

Woodman, Marion. *Addiction to Perfection: The Still Unravished Bride.* Toronto: Inner City Books, 1982.

Woodman, Marion. *The Pregnant Virgin.* Toronto: Inner City Books, 1985.

Yogendra, Sitadevi. *Yoga Physical Education for Women.* 1st ed., 1934. Mumbai: The Yoga Institute, 2008.

Yogendra, Shri. *Yoga Asanas Simplified.* 1st ed., 1928. Mumbai: The Yoga Institute, 2006.

Yong, Ed. "Why Killer Whales Go Through Menopause But Elephants Don't." *National Geographic.* March 5, 2015. https://www.nationalgeographic.com/science/phenomena/2015/03/05/why-killer-whales-go-through-menopause-but-elephants-dont/ (accessed January 17, 2019).

ABOUT THE AUTHOR

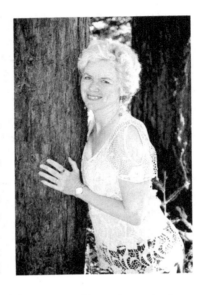

Laura Cornell (Sanskrit name Yogeshwari) is an award winning speaker, author, and sacred business mentor who helps women heal ~ body, mind, and soul ~ so they can contribute to healing the planet. She is Founder of Divine Feminine Yoga, through which she has directed seven online conferences empowering women through Yoga, and where she offers coaching, retreats, online courses and leadership training for women worldwide. It brings Laura great joy to help other women find and live their soul's purpose.

In previous work as Founder of the Green Yoga Association, Laura spurred a national movement towards Green Yoga studios and produced two major conferences on Yoga and ecology. She has been featured in Yoga Journal, Yogi Times, L.A. Yoga, and Common Ground Magazines.

Laura holds a Masters degree in East-West Psychology and a Doctorate in Religion and Philosophy. She is a certified 500-hour Kripalu Yoga teacher and Integrative Yoga Therapist. She is also a Heartfulness Meditation Practitioner. She has taught at the Kripalu Center for Yoga and Health, the Yoga Philosophy Programs of Loyola Marymount University and the California Institute for Integral Studies, the Integral Yoga Teachers Conference, and the MC Mehta Center and Mahatma Gandhi Peace Center in India.

In her 20s, Laura suffered from anxiety and depression, chronic fatigue and an eating disorder. Forging her own authentic path of healing, she discovered Yoga's transformative power to reconnect her with her feminine being and bring her home to wholeness. This book tells that story.

Made in the USA
Coppell, TX
19 June 2021

57742308R00108